HEALTH
INFORMATICS

D1584472

HEALTH INFORMATICS

A SOCIO-TECHNICAL PERSPECTIVE

SUE WHETTON

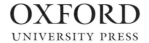

OXFORD

UNIVERSITY PRESS

253 Normanby Road, South Melbourne, Victoria 3205, Australia

Oxford University Press is a department of the University of Oxford.
It furthers the University's objective of excellence in research, scholarship,
and education by publishing worldwide in

Oxford New York

Auckland Cape Town Dar es Salaam Hong Kong Karachi
Kuala Lumpur Madrid Melbourne Mexico City Nairobi
New Delhi Shanghai Taipei Toronto

With offices in

Argentina Austria Brazil Chile Czech Republic France Greece
Guatemala Hungary Italy Japan Poland Portugal Singapore
South Korea Switzerland Thailand Turkey Ukraine Vietnam

OXFORD is a trade mark of Oxford University Press
in the UK and in certain other countries

National Library of Australia
Cataloguing-in-Publication data:

Health informatics : a socio-technical perspective.

Bibliography.
Includes index.
ISBN 0 19 555078 1.

1. Medical informatics. I. Whetton, Sue.

610.285

Typeset by Linda Hamley
Printed in Hong Kong by Sheck Wah Tong Printing Press Ltd

Contents

PART 2   HEALTH INFORMATICS TOOLS, TECHNIQUES, AND APPLICATIONS   77

4   Tools: Promises and Pitfalls   78
Sue Whetton, Chris Showell

PART 3   HEALTH INFORMATICS IN ACTION   219

Boxes

FIGURES

TABLES

Contributors

The following people made significant contributions to chapters of the book.

John D. Gillies
MB, ChB, FAAP, FRCPC, FRACP, MRSNZ

Senior Lecturer, Health Informatics, Department of Information Science, School of Business, University of Otago

John is a paediatrician in clinical practice whose interest in information management has led him to academic involvement in health informatics. He was a member of the team that established the Post Graduate Diploma in Health Informatics at the University of Otago, New Zealand. The teaching program began in 1998 and now extends to Masters and PhD informatics. The Diploma is also taught in a number of Pacific Islands. The Diploma is taught using distance learning techniques and Internet conferencing. John co-authored Chapter 8.

Jackie Hartnett
BA(Hons), M.AppComp, MACS

Lecturer, School of Computing, University of Tasmania

Jackie has been lecturing in Computer Security for the past 15 years and has a particular interest in systems that enable the confidentiality of personally identified health data to be maintained as it is shared between health care providers. In 2001 she built one of the four prototype designs for e-consent models in health for the Australian Commonwealth Government. She is also a member of several working parties for Australian standards in relation to the security of health data. Jackie assisted with security and standards content for several chapters, particularly Chapters 3 and 5.

Lauren Hoban
BA, GradDip Applied Science (Informatics)
Instructional Designer, University Department of Rural Health, Tasmania

Lauren has a background in computing and education, and has recently worked as an IT lecturer and course manager in the United Kingdom. She has extensive experience in training and assisting student, corporate, and community computer users. Lauren contributed significantly to Chapter 5.

Alec Holt
BSc, DipSci, MCom(Otago), MNZRS

Lecturer, Department of Information Science, University of Otago

Alec has received many research grants and is currently supervising twelve postgraduate students. He is listed in many international 'Who's Who' directories, has over a hundred publications, and has been an invited speaker at conferences many times. His main areas of expertise are Health Informatics, Geographical Information Systems, and Artificial Intelligence, especially case-based reasoning. He is a regular reviewer for international journals in these fields. Alec contributed to Chapter 9.

Chris Showell
B App Sci (MT), Grad Dip Prof Man

Manager, Information Systems, Hospitals and Ambulance Services Division, Tasmanian Department of Health and Human Services

Chris started working in health care part-way through the last century and has not given up yet. He has practical experience in laboratory medicine, hospital management, information systems, and health administration, and likes to 'join the dots'. He offered advice and information for several chapters, and co-authored Chapter 4.

Carol Pollard
BSc(Information systems/Computer Science), MBA, PhD (Business Administration and Management Information Systems), University of Pittsburgh

Associate Professor, School of Information Systems, University of Tasmania

Carol's research interests include decision support systems, the organisational impact of emerging technologies, the impact on workflow, the diffusion and implementation of emerging technologies, and technology transfer. Much of her current research is focused on the health care sector. A number of her research projects have received university and corporate support. Carol has published a number of articles in journals such as *MIS Quarterly*, *Journal of Management Information Systems*, *Information and Management*, *Journal of Organizational Computing*, and *International Small Business Journal* and has been invited to present her research at numerous national and international conferences. She has consulted to a number of private and not-for-profit organisations on the training and deployment of decision support systems and the evaluation, selection, and implementation of emerging technologies. She served as the Executive Secretary of ICIS from 1995 to 1999 and is currently Adviser Director of SIGGROUP for the Association of Computing Machinery, Vice President of the International Global Information Technology Management Association, and Conference Chair for the 15th Annual Australasian Conference on Information Systems. Carol co-authored Chapters 6 and 9.

Judi Walker
BA (Hons) Grad Dip Ed MACE PhD

Professor of Rural Health, Associate Dean, Teaching and Learning, Deputy Dean, Faculty of Health Sciences, University of Tasmania

Judi holds the inaugural Chair of Rural Health at the University of Tasmania and has overall responsibility for the Faculty of Health Science's academic rural health portfolio. She is Chief Executive of the University's Rural Clinical School, which is a conjoint appointment with the Tasmanian Department of Health and Human Services. Judi sits on the editorial boards of a number of international journals and publishes widely. She is recognised for her scholarship and related academic activities in rural health, primary health care, and medical education. She is Acting Chair of the Tasmania Together Progress Board and is a member of the Australian Ambulance Education Council. Recently she was appointed to the NHMRC Training Awards Committee. Judi co-authored Chapter 10.

Hugh J. Watson
BS (Electrical Engineering), MBA (Management), DBA (Management)

Professor of Management Information Systems, Terry College of Business, University of Georgia; holder of a C. Herman and Mary Virginia Terry Chair of Business Administration

Hugh is one of the world's leading scholars and authorities on decision support. He is the author of twenty-two books and over a hundred scholarly journal articles. He helped develop much of the conceptual foundation for decision support systems in the 1970s and applied his knowledge and expertise to executive information systems in the 1980s. Hugh is recognised as a leader in the academic community. He was conference chair for DSS-90, program chair for the 1995 Association for Information Systems conference, and serves on the Hawaii International Conference on System Sciences executive committee. He was elected to the Decision Sciences Institute's Executive Council, served on the organising committee for the Association for Information Systems (AIS), was elected as an AIS Americas Region Council Member, and was twice a candidate for AIS president. Hugh offered an invaluable review of Chapter 9.

Sue Whetton
BA, Dip T(P), Dip Cont Ed, MIS

Lecturer, Online Educational Development, University Department of Rural Health, and, Deputy Associate Dean, Teaching and Learning, Faculty of Health Services, University of Tasmania.

Sue established and currently coordinates the Department's E-Health Graduate Program, which utilises a unique pathway concept to facilitate different learning styles and different skill levels. Her varied career includes teaching, working with disadvantaged groups, lecturing in sociology, and working as an independent consultant. Sue has published and presented at conferences in both health informatics and flexible education. She is currently studying for her PhD, exploring the influence of discourses on the emergence of health informatics as a discipline and a profession. Sue is the primary author and content editor for this text.

Brendon J. Woodford
BSc, DipSc, MSc

Lecturer and Senior Member, Knowledge Intelligence and Web Informatics (KIWI) Lab, Department of Information Science, University of Otago

Brendon's current research interests include image processing and image recognition, knowledge discovery from connectionist-based systems, fuzzy systems design and development, data mining, and advanced data visualisation techniques. He is currently pursuing a PhD in the area of applying connectionist-based intelligent information systems for knowledge discovery in horticulture. Brendon provided invaluable advice and resources for Chapter 9.

Preface

Health informatics is a multi-disciplinary, multi-dimensional field that seeks to facilitate the effective collection, management and use of information in the health care environment. By its very nature, health informatics is challenging and complex. Yet it is this complexity that makes it such an intriguing, exciting, and rewarding field in which to be involved. This book introduces the field of health informatics.

The book adopts a socio-technical perspective. A socio-technical perspective, while exploring the technical aspects of health informatics, focuses on the interplay between the health care environment and the systems used to manage information in that environment. Such a perspective enables analysis of the complex health care environment with its many different service systems and professional groups, each with their own ideas and views about health matters, including health informatics. One of the challenges for the health informatics professional is to identify and seek to accommodate these different views. The socio-technical focus of the book facilitates this by encouraging the reader to ask questions such as:

- Who are the key players?
- How will the introduction of this system affect key players?
- How will key players view the introduction of this system?
- How do we balance the interests of key players?

Adopting a socio-technical perspective encourages the reader to consider the potential impact of health informatics systems on the health care environment. While the aim is for more effective management of information, it is widely acknowledged that health informatics has the capacity to do more than simply slot into the existing environment. It has the potential to be a catalyst for dramatic change, cutting across traditional structures, roles, processes and relationships, and influencing the way health systems are organised and delivered. This textbook explores the potential for key players to use health informatics to reshape the health care environment by tackling questions such as:

- What is the potential impact of health informatics on the structure and delivery of health care?

- How does the introduction of health informatics systems and technologies impact on the traditional authority, roles, and relationships of health care professionals and consumers?
- Who will be the main beneficiaries of this system?
- How will this system enable consumers to receive better health care and at what cost will this be achieved?

The book has been influenced by the concerns and focus of health informatics itself. While exploring practical applications, it also investigates the scope and distinguishing features of the discipline. Thus, it acknowledges that the health informatics community consists of a diverse mix of academics and practitioners who, while sharing the goal of enhancing health care, may identify different issues, priorities, and approaches for achieving these. This text encourages students to identify and critique these different perspectives.

A fundamental premise of the book is that the promise of health informatics will be realised more readily if we understand the different perspectives of the key players and their ability to shape both the discipline and its practical applications. Therefore, as the theory and application of health informatics are explored, underlying questions are:

- What are the questions and issues addressed?
- Which key player perspective does this represent?
- What alternative perspectives can be identified?
- Do these alternatives point to different questions and issues?
- How do we balance these different views?

WHO IS THIS BOOK FOR?

Since this book seeks to present a range of stakeholder perspectives, it can be used by different health professional and consumer groups as an introduction to the field. Intending health informatics professionals can use the book to develop their skills and knowledge. At the same time, since health informatics is a multi-disciplinary field, the intending health informatics professional will want to seek out additional specialist resources on specific topics.

Think of the text as a beach, with a particular feature being the exploration of health informatics from a socio-cultural perspective. Practising health professionals and consumers may wish to paddle around in the shallower waters, occasionally venturing out into deeper water to explore areas of specific interest. The intending health informatics professional will want to wade out into the deeper water, spend a lot of time swimming around a wide area, perhaps doing a little snorkelling to explore the features in greater detail. He or she will eventually move on to other beaches with different features.

ORGANISATION OF THE BOOK

The book is organised into three parts:
* Foundations of Health Informatics
* Health Informatics Tools, Techniques, and Applications
* Health Informatics in Action.

Part 1: Foundations of Health Informatics

The first part of the book introduces and explores health informatics from a socio-cultural perspective. Our understanding of health informatics as a discipline and a profession will be enhanced by understanding the social context within which it is located. Chapter 1 explores the dynamics between health informatics and the socio-cultural environment of health. Chapter 2 focuses on the emerging discipline of health informatics, exploring the parameters of the discipline and its subsets. Chapter 3 discusses key concepts and theories used to develop the knowledge base and inform the practice of health informatics.

Part 2: Health Informatics Tools, Techniques and Applications

The second part focuses on the tools and techniques of health informatics. Chapter 4 reviews current hardware, software, and communications technologies, identifying issues around the use of these in the health care environment. Chapters 5 and 6 discuss key concepts and principles of data collection and information management and apply these to the health environment. Chapters 7, 8, and 9 explore e-health, electronic health records, and decision support systems, which are currently the focus of much activity. A number of yet-to-be-resolved issues are identified and the reader is encouraged to critically evaluate the vision and the realities of these various applications.

Part 3: Health Informatics in Action

The last part is a discussion of health informatics in action. It consists of one chapter, which explores the use of health informatics in the rural and remote health care environment.

Acknowledgments

There are a number of people who must be thanked for their contributions, advice and feedback throughout the writing of this book. For their assistance with examples, illustrations, and case studies, my thanks to Lisa Dalton, John Gillies, Alec Holt, Emily Mauldon, and Julia Monaghan. For critical reviews, editing, feedback, and advice, my thanks to Daphne Habibis, Lauren Hoban, Karla Peek, Tina Pinkard, and Karen Willis, and to Eva Murray for invaluable research assistance.

Acronyms

AMIA	American Medical Informatics Association
COACH	Canada's Health Informatics Association
CIO	chief information officer
CDSS	clinical decision support systems
CKO	chief knowledge officer
DSS	decision support system
HINZ	Health Informatics New Zealand
HISA	Health Informatics Society of Australia
IDS	intrusion detection system
IMIA	International Medical Informatics Association
IT	information technology
ICTs	information and communication technologies
LAN	local area network
PID	personally identifiable data
PII	personally identified information
RAD	rapid applications development
RISP	Regional Information Systems Plan
SDLC	systems development life cycle
WAN	wide area network
WHO	World Health Organization
WWW	World Wide Web
UKCHIP	United Kingdom Council for Health Informatics Professions

PART 1

FOUNDATIONS OF HEALTH INFORMATICS

Most people interested in health informatics just want to *do it*. That is, they want to be involved in planning, designing, developing, and using **health information systems** and applications.

Unfortunately, health informatics operates within the health environment, which is inherently political and made up of a complex mix of people, **organisations**, and technology. Health care is resource intensive, and no health care system today has sufficient resources to provide a comprehensive and complete service. This means that decisions have to be made at the political, organisational, and individual level regarding the allocation of those resources that are available. This gives rise to factions, pressure groups, and interest groups, who lobby both in the wider environment and within specific health care systems. The first part of this book explores this social and political context of health informatics.

CHAPTER 1

THE HEALTH CARE ENVIRONMENT AND HEALTH INFORMATICS

OVERVIEW

The complex, hierarchical health care systems established during the twentieth century are finding it increasingly difficult to provide the level of care expected by **health consumers** in the twenty-first century. Many of the challenges they face originate in the way these systems have traditionally provided services and managed the ever-increasing amounts of **information** generated in the process. Many services and systems are inappropriate for the contemporary health environment with its changing demographics and medical problems, and its emphasis on consumer-centred service delivery, continuity of care across services, **evidence-based practice,** and the shift of resources and services beyond traditional hospital-based care into community care and preventative programs. New approaches need to be developed and the emerging discipline of health informatics is widely viewed as the means for achieving this. Yet, as health informatics is introduced into the health care environment, we are realising that the changes that occur have the potential to challenge many of the assumptions and structures underpinning traditional health care.

OBJECTIVES

At the completion of this chapter, you should be able to:
- identify influences shaping the biomedical model of health
- discuss challenges faced by the traditional biomedical model
- outline the potential for health informatics to resolve some of these problems
- discuss the potential for health informatics to reinvent health care.

CONCEPTS

Worldview	Socio-technical
Globalisation	Biomedicine
Bureaucracy	Technocentric

INTRODUCTION

This chapter establishes the context for an exploration of the discipline and practice of health informatics. It does so by focusing on the characteristics of contemporary health systems in developed nations, the forces that shaped them, and the issues they currently face. The expectation that health informatics will resolve many of these problems is explored. The discussion then moves beyond this expectation to consider the proposition that health informatics can be a catalyst for reinventing health care.

Great expectations

> Throughout the late 20th century the experience of technological 'progress' and a sense of it being unstoppable, has given rise to a belief in both its inevitability and desirability, with positive consequences in societal and organisational terms (Cornford & Klecun-Dabrowska 2003, p. 353).

Since the late twentieth century there has been widespread optimism that information and communications technologies can 'break down barriers', 'transcend national, geographic and social boundaries', 'bring economic growth and prosperity' and generally enrich the lives of individuals and communities around the world. 'From trade to telemedicine, from education to environmental protection, we have in our hands, on our desktops and in the skies above, the ability to improve standards of living for millions upon millions of people' (Annan 2003, p. 1).

Those involved in the provision of health services shared this optimism. The emerging field of health informatics was viewed as the means for resolving many of the problems beginning to plague health services. These expectations were not unfounded. As Box 1.1 illustrates, success stories were told.

BOX 1.1

EARLY SUCCESSES

- Garvan-ESI was an **expert system** developed in 1984 at the Garvan Institute of Medical Research, St Vincent's Hospital, Sydney. It was used to assist with the interpretation of tests for thyroid levels and was said to be 99 per cent accurate.
- One of the first computer-based medical records systems was the HELP system used by the LDS Hospital in Salt Lake City from 1975. A version of this system was still being used in 1998.

Yet, as seen in Box 1.2, there are also numerous stories of projects unfinished, unused, or unable to fulfil expectations.

There are undoubtedly more examples of what could be considered failures than there are successes. This might suggest that the promise of health informatics has not been fulfilled, and that expectations were too high. But perhaps this is not the case.

BOX 1.2

SOMETHING WENT WRONG

- Introduced on 26 October 1992, the London Ambulance Service Computer Aided Despatch (LASCAD) system included a tracking system, communications system, a database, and a map-based display interface. The system was supposed to automate the deployment of London ambulances to ensure that emergency calls were answered with minimum waiting time. After two days of operation the system response time began to slow down until it finally locked up altogether on 4 November.

- In 1985, the Regional Information Systems Plan (RISP) of Wessex Health Authority, England, began operation. The Authority aimed to install computer terminals in all offices, hospitals, and wards in the region. When RISP was abandoned in 1990, only a ledger system had been provided in every district. There were accounts systems in five districts, and one hospital had implemented the hospital information system.

Perhaps we simply did not adequately understand all the issues involved in the introduction of health informatics systems into the health care environment.

Early approaches to health informatics mirrored those of business and commerce, concentrating on designing information systems to automate existing manual tasks and **workflows** in administrative and financial areas. Interest focused on technology such as hardware requirements and capabilities, software design, systems development, and algorithmic problem solving. There was little interest in organisational and cultural factors. It was assumed that information technology would easily slot into the health environment and be enthusiastically adopted by the 'user'.

This approach, today described as **technocentric**, worked relatively well for business processes, which were and continue to be 'the most fully developed component of health informatics' (Delucca & Enmark 2000, p. 5). In the clinical environment, however, acceptance of health informatics has been slower. Hindsight suggests that the technocentric approach, 'dominated by data driven methodologies, tools and techniques that produce technical solutions to organisational problems' (Atkinson et al. 2001, p. 1), has been a significant factor.

We now understand that while technical issues are an integral element of the health informatics domain, we must move beyond these to explore organisational and cultural factors. This has led to the adoption of a **socio-technical** perspective incorporating organisational and cultural analyses with the more traditional computing and information systems tools and processes. Adopting this perspective has broadened our thinking about the potential of health informatics. It has taken us beyond the view that information technologies will slot neatly into the existing health care environment. Today we realise that health informatics has the potential to support dramatic and widespread changes to these structures and processes: 'The emergence of new information and communication technologies…is often seen as offering new opportunities for enhanced levels of care, structural reform and organisational modernisation in health care' (Cornford & Klecun-Dabrowska 2003, p. 343).

The opportunity for dramatic change is increasingly viewed as essential for the viability of health services in the future (Berwick 2002, Cornford & Klecun-Dabrowska. 2003). It is a view shared by health professionals and consumers alike. A 1998 survey of patient satisfaction, sponsored by the Harvard School of Public Health, found that in each of three countries—the USA, Canada, and Australia—79 per cent of the population said their system needs either 'fundamental change' or to be 'completely rebuilt'. The same sentiment was expressed by 89 per cent in New Zealand and by 72 per cent in the United Kingdom (National Centre for Policy Analysis 2000).

The starting point for understanding this view, and the expectations for health informatics, is to consider contemporary health systems, the influences that shaped them and the challenges they face today.

CONTEMPORARY HEALTH SYSTEMS

Health care today, particularly in advanced industrial nations, is widely described as a system—a complex, often cumbersome mix of community- and hospital-based services, provided by a bewildering array of health professionals located in public and private facilities and organisations across the country. Individual nations have their own arrangements for funding these systems, for insuring consumers, and for reimbursing health professionals. They differ in the mix of public, private, and not-for-profit services, and have different mechanisms by which patients locate, select, and access services. Box 1.3 provides an overview of the arrangements for five health care systems. For more information, refer to the WWW links at the end of this chapter.

BOX 1.3

STRUCTURE OF CONTEMPORARY HEALTH CARE SYSTEMS

Australia

The Australian Medicare system provides free access to public hospital services and assists with the cost of a range of medical services. Private health insurance is available to assist with costs relating to private patients in private and public hospitals and for services not covered by Medicare. The Commonwealth has a **role** in policy development, research funding, and national and international health issues. States and Territories manage public health services, deliver public acute care, psychiatric hospital services, and community and public health. The majority of doctors and many allied health professionals are self-employed. Private hospitals are owned by both for-profit and not-for-profit organisations.

Canada

The Canadian system provides universal access to hospital inpatient, out-patient, and physician services. The majority of these services are privately delivered but publicly funded. There is no significant private health sector. Responsibility for health services is shared between provincial and federal governments. The federal government collects taxes, allocates funds to provinces, sets **standards** and guidelines, and takes responsibility for health promotion, illness prevention, education, and research. Provincial governments manage and deliver health services, planning, financing, and evaluating hospital care, physician and allied health care services, and public health.

New Zealand

The New Zealand system is based around publicly funded universal access to secondary health care. The government allocates money to District Health Boards, who are responsible for the purchase of health services. The government provides broad guidelines about the services that the Boards must provide. Boards contract public, private, and voluntary organisations to provide services. Primary care services are not publicly funded. There is a subsidy for primary care costs for those on low incomes. Private health insurance assists with the cost of private services such as private hospitals, laboratories, radiology centres, medical specialists, and general practitioners.

United Kingdom

In the United Kingdom, health care is funded and provided by the government and all residents have equal access to medical services. The National Health Service (NHS) is responsible for strategic planning, while Strategic Health Authorities plan and provide primary and secondary health care for the region they cover. Primary services are provided locally. More specialised services such as hospitals, ambulances, and specialised health services are provided in fewer locations. There is also a small private health insurance system.

USA

The US government provides a means-tested safety net system for those on low incomes and free basic cover for the elderly and people with disabilities. For the general community, the US system is based on private health insurance provided by for-profit and not-for-profit companies. These are regulated by State governments, which are also responsible for planning the provision of hospitals and nursing homes. Insurance packages vary considerably in terms of the coverage offered. Many health care organisations, including hospitals and nursing homes, are for-profit companies. There are also some not-for-profit hospitals and government-run hospitals.

These different arrangements impact on the issues and solutions, including health information management issues and solutions, within each health system. Yet despite the unique social, political, and economic circumstances that gave rise to these individual arrangements, the systems also share a number of common characteristics. Since they evolved within the industrial societies of the twentieth century, all were subject to the same or similar ideas and influences. The fundamental influence was the scientific view of the world.

Scientific view of the world

> It is our culture's beliefs and values that shape what we will create and what we dream (Coiera 2004, p. 5).

Underpinning every society is a view of the world, which provides explanations for physical and social phenomena, shapes social institutions, and influences how people interact with one another. In Western Europe prior to the sixteenth century, religious thinking and religious institutions dominated: 'Answers to questions about existence were found from within the body of Christian **knowledge** and most social institutions were also closely tied to the church' (van Krieken et al. 2000, p. 23).

Within this **worldview**, illness was often interpreted as divine retribution or the work of the devil, and prayer and religious beliefs played an integral role in treatment and recovery. These explanations were not able to be objectively verified, but were accepted on faith.

The nineteenth and twentieth centuries were characterised by a more secular worldview based on rational, scientific thinking. Within this worldview the physical and social world was seen as structured by universal laws that linked events together in cause-and-effect relationships. Rational science sought to identify these relationships and laws. As new relationships and laws were identified, so knowledge was created. The scientific worldview stressed the objective nature of the world. Knowledge was valid only if it was observed through the senses.

Rational science viewed illness as the result of identifiable organic or physical phenomena. Application of the scientific method would identify the cause, enabling diagnosis, treatment, and a cure. This was a very appealing worldview since it included the assumption that we are not subject to the caprices of an unpredictable deity. If the world is ordered by cause-and-effect relationships, and we can identify these, then we can have some influence on events.

Science, with its emphasis on logic and rationality, influenced Western thinking throughout the nineteenth and twentieth centuries. It shaped ideas about what type of knowledge is important and about how that knowledge is created and used. It also influenced the way Western societies structure their social organisations and relationships.

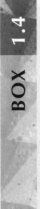

BOX 1.4

WORLDVIEWS AND EXPLANATIONS OF DISEASE: AN EXAMPLE

A mysterious disease sweeps through the community. Entire households fall ill and many die. In sixteenth-century Europe, the religious world-view attributes the disease as a punishment from God, resulting in prayers and possibly donations to the church. As the disease peters out, the community thanks God for sparing them and vows to sin no more. In contemporary Australia, the scientific worldview assumes that this is a highly contagious bacterial or viral infection. Victims and their immediate family may be quarantined to prevent further spread of the disease, while biomedical scientists identify the cause, develop a cure, and produce a vaccine to protect people in the future. Once the disease is controlled, the scientists are recognised in the Australia Day honours list and a pharmaceutical company takes out a copyright on the vaccine.

The scientific worldview in practice

Ideas emerging from the scientific worldview included:

- Scientific knowledge is superior to non-scientific knowledge.
- Scientific knowledge is cumulative.
- Science and knowledge equal progress.
- Rationalism as an effective means for structuring organisations.

Scientific knowledge rules!

The dominance of the scientific worldview in Western thinking has seen scientific knowledge generally holding a higher **status** than non-rational forms of knowledge. Those who possess scientific knowledge often hold a higher status in the community. In the health environment, those with scientific medical knowledge are perceived as more knowledgeable than those trained in traditional or alternative therapies. By the middle of the twentieth century, very few people considered consulting anyone other than a registered clinician who practiced science-based medicine.

Scientific knowledge grows

Scientific knowledge is cumulative. It is created by building on existing knowledge. As it grows it differentiates and becomes increasingly specialised. To manage this, new disciplines and professions emerge. The many health specialties and subspecialties are a result of increased **differentiation** of biomedical knowledge.

The growth of scientific knowledge during the last few decades has been so rapid that we are now living in what has been defined as the information age. Health, with its ever-expanding biomedical knowledge base and increasing amounts of **data** and information required for day-to-day service delivery, epitomises the information age. The need to efficiently manage health information has given rise to the discipline of health informatics.

Science and technology equal progress

The belief that science enables us to influence our social and physical world resulted in scientific development being widely viewed as synonymous with progress, and progress is widely viewed as desirable. The discovery of penicillin, the ability to perform organ transplants, and the eradication of smallpox are examples of progress arising from rational science.

Since science and technology are often linked together in twentieth-century thinking, technological development is also widely viewed as synonymous with progress. In health care, science and technology have enabled the development of increasingly sophisticated interventions and treatments, an expanding array of pharmaceuticals, complex tests and analyses, and ever more sophisticated surgical techniques. Many of us today view the use of advanced medical treatments and technologies as synonymous with high quality care.

Bureaucracy is ideal

The scientific worldview shaped many aspects of twentieth-century society. Of particular relevance to health care is the application of rationalism and differentiation to the structure of organisations. The most common form of organisation in contemporary Western society is the **bureaucracy**, which has been described as 'the ultimate manifestation of rationality in social organisation' (Bilton et al 1996, p. 38). Bureaucracies divide work tasks and responsibilities into hierarchically organised, specialised departments and sections. Apart from very small practices, health services have typically adopted rational bureaucratic structures that organise a range of clinicians, administrators, managers, and other support professionals into a hierarchy of roles, statuses, and responsibilities.

Globalisation: other ways of thinking

Globalisation is a phenomenom closely linked to science and progress. It is a process that has been occurring for several decades as the economic, political, and cultural aspects of communities become increasingly interconnected. Advances in communications technology in the 1990s accelerated the process. Networks such as the Internet now enable the instant communication and exchange of information across the globe. While many view globalisation as a positive development, it is resulting in some new health issues. Box 1.5 lists some of these.

Efforts to deal with the problems arising from globalisation are bringing about increased cooperation between national governments and international organisations,

BOX 1.5

GLOBALISATION CREATES NEW HEALTH ISSUES

- Increased health risks from the spread of infectious diseases, and biological and chemical terrorism arising from increased international commerce, tourist, and refugee movements.
- Small, locally managed health services and businesses being absorbed into large, national, and trans-national organisations, which are difficult for national authorities to monitor and regulate.
- Globalisation of Western popular **culture** and lifestyles, resulting in the globalisation of **diseases of affluence**—heart disease, obesity, and diabetes.
- Migration of health professionals from developing countries, resulting in increasing health inequities between developed and developing nations.

such as the World Health Organization (WHO), and the collection and exchange of information across State and national boundaries is integral to these efforts.

Globalisation has also exposed Western societies to different ways of thinking. This is generating discussion, including the suggestion that reality is more complex than the sensory-based, factual view presented by rational science. There is increasing discussion about the legitimacy of non-sensory, intuitive knowledge in many areas of social life, including health: 'Although the biomedical model of disease and its associated professional and institutional forms remains dominant in modern society, it is increasingly coming under scrutiny and attack' (van Krieken et al 2000, p. 173).

Exposure to these alternative worldviews has led, in the West, to renewed interest in the mind and body relationship in health and illness. Many people are turning to alternative therapies and traditional practices. These include homoeopathy, chiropractic treatments, traditional Chinese medicine, meditation, and the traditional belief systems of indigenous peoples.

These alternative views are combining with the knowledge and processes of **biomedicine** to shape contemporary health systems and the issues they face.

Contemporary health systems: shared characteristics

Characteristics of health systems in developed nations include:

- the knowledge- and technology-intensive biomedical model
- specialisation and differentiation
- bureaucratic structures
- health care structured around the face-to-face consultation.

Technology-intensive biomedical model

> The central knowledge base of modern medical science is usually known as biomedicine (van Krieken et al. 2000, p. 142).

Biomedicine attributes disease to physical causes such as viruses and bacteria, and uses scientific method to identify the causes and treat the diseases. Biomedicine began to gain ascendancy in the early nineteenth century when control of infectious diseases was a priority, when many chronic or non-communicable conditions were difficult to treat, and when hospital care was generally for the more seriously and acutely ill. Biomedical health systems therefore tended to focus on acute health issues, with hospitals as the centre of care, while preventative care, community education, and other services were placed in an ancillary role.

Over the last hundred years improved living standards and medical advances have led to a decrease in infectious diseases, an increase in successful interventions for formerly untreatable conditions, and, in many countries, an increased life expectancy. The biomedical model is generally viewed as having contributed to these better health and medical outcomes through the use of increasingly complex tests and treatments. Unfortunately, as Table 1.1 shows, these treatments and technologies are demanding more and more resources each year and many nations are unable, or unwilling, to continue allocating ever-greater resources to seemingly insatiable health systems.

Table 1.1 Health expenditure as percentage of gross domestic product 1997–2001

Country	1997	1998	1999	2000	2001
Australia	8.5	8.6	8.7	8.9	9.2
Canada	8.9	9.1	9.1	9.1	9.5
New Zealand	7.5	7.9	8	8	8.3
United Kingdom	6.8	6.9	7.2	7.3	7.6
USA	13	13	13	13.1	13.9

Source: adapted from the World Health Report 2004 Changing History.

At the same time, recent trends, at least at the policy level, have shown a shift away from the traditional hospital-centred focus of biomedicine and an increasing emphasis on community-based service delivery, disease prevention, health-promotion activities, and on involving patients as active partners in their care. Box 1.6 illustrates these changes in policy.

These trends, together with the increasing use of alternative therapies and practices, reflect the alternative worldviews that began to influence our thinking in the last decades of the twentieth century. 'There is a shifting paradigm from the costly illness-centered, hospital-based care, to community-based care with an emphasis on health promotion and disease prevention' (Duffett-Leger 1996, p. 1).

BOX 1.6

THE CHANGING FOCUS OF HEALTH CARE

Australia

The National Health Priority Areas (NHPA) initiative...recognises that specific strategies for reducing the burden of illness should be holistic, encompassing the continuum of care from health promotion and illness prevention, through to treatment and management (Commonwealth Department of Health and Family Services 1998, p. 6).

Canada

Ministers recognise that improving access to care will require...strategic investments in areas such as: increasing the supply of health professionals; effective community-based services, including home care; a pharmaceuticals strategy; effective health promotion and disease prevention, and adequate financial resources (Office of the Prime Minister 2004).

New Zealand

This principle reflects the Government's desire to have a health system that promotes good health and 'wellness' as well as treating illness. Many of the illnesses affecting the New Zealand population are potentially preventable, and we need to do better at addressing all the determinants of health (New Zealand Ministry of Health 2000, p. 1).

United Kingdom

A key is...using more sophisticated methods to get the right messages to the right target groups and individuals...a focus on supporting and encouraging people to choose how they look after themselves...It is about self-awareness of symptoms and taking specific actions to monitor one's own well-being as well as making lifestyle changes (UK Department of Health 2001).

USA

We are encouraging American families to take small, manageable steps within their current lifestyle to ensure long-term health...Improve health literacy: ability of an individual to access, understand, and use health-related information and services to make appropriate health decisions (Office of the Surgeon General 2004).

Specialisation and differentiation of health professions

The differentiation of biomedicine into specialties and subspecialties has created professional groups with strong cultures and clearly delineated roles, relationships, and professional boundaries, which are organised into an identifiable status hierarchy. Medical doctors, traditionally viewed as possessing the most medical knowledge, are usually accorded the highest status. Other medical and health professions are situated in the hierarchy according to their perceived level or type of scientific knowledge. Some professional groups have guarded their areas of expertise carefully, resulting in the emergence of professional **silos**. 'Specialist silo systems serve to contain and isolate. Each specialty has its own body of workers, is sustained by its own agenda, and drives its own research programs, the outcomes of which are discussed at specialist meetings and published in specialist journals' (Chew & Van Der Weyden 2002, p. 20).

This professional differentiation emerged in and was maintained by the traditional biomedical system where patients were passed backwards and forwards along the chain of health professionals for one-to-one consultations and treatment. Current trends, including interdisciplinary care, community-based care, and the involvement of patients in decision-making, together with the introduction of information and communications systems, are challenging specialist silos and the associated roles and relationships, creating new linkages and opportunities for communication and collaboration. Box 1.7 shows how a videoconference can foster these changes.

BOX 1.7 RELATIONSHIPS AND INTERACTION IN A VIDEO CONSULTATION

A video consultation may involve a specialist in a major urban hospital, a community nurse, general practitioner, or other health professional, and the patient in a rural location. The consultation becomes a collaborative process, as participants share information and discussion. This contrasts with the traditional process where the information and the patient were passed along the chain for one-to-one consultations. It facilitates a more equal relationship among health professionals and between health professionals and consumers.

Bureaucratic structures

A significant percentage of today's health services continue to be offered within large, complex and hierarchical organisations. Managing these organisations has given rise to complex, status hierarchies and **power** structures. Van Krieken et al. (2000) refer to a 'dual structure' with bureaucratic/managerial personnel on the one hand, and medical personnel on the other. Status hierarchies and power structures are even more complex today. One example is the emergence of departments of information management with their own agendas and their own specific knowledge domain. An indication of the importance of information in today's health systems is seen in the status and power held by many Chief Information Officers (CIO) or Chief Knowledge Officers. These positions are often located at senior management level and add an additional dimension to the hierarchies and power relationships.

Another example is the creation of new positions such as clinical managers, which were created to involve clinicians more directly in management processes. These positions were intended to facilitate increased understanding and cooperation between managers and clinicians. Research suggests, however, that such positions exacerbate existing tensions between both clinical specialties and clinicians and management (Degeling et al 2003, Forbes et al 2004, Lemioux-Charles et al 1993, Willcocks 2004). Findings relating to clinical managers, include:

- The attitudes of different professions towards involvement in the management process are shaped, at least in part, by perceptions of increased opportunities and status vis-à-vis other professions.
- Clinical managers often experience conflict as they try to balance decisions about financial and human resources with their professional commitment to high quality care.
- Clinical mangers often find themselves viewed with suspicion by both clinicians and managers: 'I get accused with the management team of being a doctor and my colleagues hate me because I am a manager...it's like being Head boy, you can't win' (Willcocks 2004).

While management structures within larger health facilities are becoming increasingly complex, the trend towards community-based, interdisciplinary care has seen some facilities develop flatter management structures with increased opportunity for participation in decision-making. This trend is creating new linkages and relationships. Box 1.8 illustrates the changes occurring between health professionals and patients.

Health care structured around the face-to-face consultation

Throughout most of the twentieth century, interaction between health professionals and their patients was based around the face-to-face consultation. As the health professional,

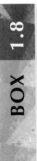

THE CONSUMER AS PARTNER

BOX 1.8

Health consumers (who used to be patients) have generally been located at the lower levels of the hierarchy. The professional, as the possessor of knowledge, has been the senior partner in the relationship. An increasing emphasis on community-based care, health promotion, and disease prevention in recent years has seen patients and their families becoming more involved in decision-making. As a result, there is growing dissatisfaction with the 'professional as expert' approach. Patients and their families are beginning to seek involvement on a more equal basis.

usually the family doctor, gathered information from the patient, a relationship of trust was built up. This relationship was highly valued and the face-to-face consultation is still considered by many to be a central component of effective health care.

This model emerged early in the twentieth century when the family doctor provided the bulk of health and medical care, and referrals for tests and specialist services were the exception rather than the **norm**. The consultation was the primary source for information gathering, and for the dispensing of care and treatment. In today's health environment, the first point of contact for health issues continues to be the general practitioner, community nurse, or other primary care professional. However, referrals for tests, examinations, or additional consultations are now commonplace. Since significant information is acquired from these sources, there is an argument that the face-to-face consultation is no longer the primary source of information gathering.

While the number and variety of health professionals we interact with has increased, so too have the demands on the time of health professionals. This also puts pressure on the centrality of the face-to-face encounter. Although it continues to be seen as an integral element of health care, the reality is that it has become increasingly difficult to maintain.

CHALLENGES FOR CONTEMPORARY HEALTH CARE SYSTEMS

The structure and processes of contemporary health care have enhanced the ability of health services to offer high quality care and improve health outcomes for many individuals. At the same time they have created challenges relating to:

- meeting demand
- managing the resulting information.

Meeting demand

Health care is resource intensive and no health system today has sufficient resources to provide a comprehensive and complete service. Demands on resources include the following:

- Individuals spend longer in the health system and consume more health resources than ever before due to the increasing use of diagnostic tests and other specialist services.
- The complexities of health systems have seen large, complex, and unwieldy organisations emerge. Managing these requires an ever-increasing percentage of health resources.
- Changes in disease patterns in Western populations have seen cardiovascular diseases, stress-related diseases, diabetes, and obesity becoming major health problems. Treatment for these conditions often requires the expensive complex technology, skilled clinicians, and ongoing treatment, which are currently creating resourcing issues for many health services.

- Western societies have ageing populations. While not all older people require health care, as the population ages, demands for health care will increase, as older people often have multiple health issues and higher support needs.
- Globalisation is seeing national, state, and local health authorities increasingly required to implement systems and strategies to deal with health problems associated with global epidemics and the threat of terrorist attacks.

These developments are placing considerable stresses on our traditional systems, and demand is currently outstripping our ability to provide services. Resources are being rationed and decisions to fund some services and facilities are often made at the expense of others.

Hospital executives responding to the 2003 Commonwealth Fund International Health Policy Survey believed that inadequate funding and staffing shortages would be the two biggest problems faced by hospitals in the next decade (see Table 1.2). The different priorities identified by hospital executives in each country illustrate the influence of the different funding, insurance, and service-delivery arrangements discussed earlier.

Table 1.2 Two biggest problems faced by hospitals

Per cent naming	Australia	Canada	New Zealand	United Kingdom	USA
Inadequate funding	58	62	57	39	10
Inadequate reimbursement	8	—	—	—	60
Staffing shortage	45	60	54	64	47
Inadequate/overcrowded or outdated facilities	32	39	54	42	7
Indigent care/uninsured	—	—	—	—	17
Malpractice costs	6	—	—	—	11

Commonwealth Fund 2003 International Survey of Hospital Executives, used with permission.

Managing health information

The biomedical model generates ever-increasing amounts of information. This includes both the biomedical knowledge base, which informs professional practice, and administrative information generated in the day-to-day operation of health services. The need to effectively manage this information is a significant challenge today, and technology is increasingly being viewed as a means of meeting this challenge.

Biomedical information

Traditionally, health professionals relied on their acquired knowledge, experience, and common sense for clinical practice. Rare or unusual problems were solved by consulting textbooks or colleagues, while new knowledge was accessed through professional journals, conferences, and books. This was a perfectly adequate approach for many decades. Today, however, the sheer volume of information creates difficulties for health professionals. Textbooks quickly become dated and colleagues might give many different answers to the same question. Coiera (2003, p. xxii) goes so far as to suggest that the amount of information being generated has placed the scientific method itself under threat: 'As medical research ploughs ahead in laboratories and clinics across the world, like some great theory machine, medical practitioners are being swamped by its results...So health care workers find themselves unable, even if they had the time, to keep abreast of the knowledge of best practice hidden in that literature.'

Day-to-day management and access

In the day-to-day operation of health services, a great deal of health-related information is generated about organisations, departments, health professionals, and consumers. This includes personal and clinical information pertaining to individual patients as well as administrative, financial, and management information relating to the organisation. This information needs to be stored securely but made accessible to relevant individuals and organisations. The amount of information generated, and the number of individuals needing (or seeking) access, continues to increase, as does the number of locations where information is stored. The increasing interconnectedness of contemporary health systems means that much more of this information is now available to many more individuals within and across organisations. Access, **security**, and **confidentiality** are thus significant problems.

Enter health informatics

> Health informatics is....concerned with the collection, storage, retrieval, communication and optimal use of health related data, information and knowledge (HISA 2004).

Many challenges facing contemporary health care systems originate in the way the systems have traditionally provided services and managed the ever-increasing amounts of information generated in the process. These methods are inappropriate for the contemporary health environment with its emphasis on consumer-centred service delivery, continuity of care across services, evidence-based practice, and the shift of resources and services beyond traditional hospital-based care into community care and preventative programs. We need to find new ways of structuring services and managing the information generated. And so we arrive once more at our great expectations for health informatics.

GREAT EXPECTATIONS REVISITED

While health informatics has been a presence in the health environment for several decades, and many projects can claim at least some measure of success, if we were to ask the question today, 'How much difference has health informatics made in solving the wider problems faced by contemporary health care services?', the answer would have to be, 'Overall, not a great deal'.

Discrete projects

Health informatics programs have had a limited impact, partly because the majority of early projects were discrete, short term, and ad hoc. This is not surprising. Health informatics applications (as with any new development) must prove their worth. Health organisations are reluctant to invest significant resources in untried systems. Thus, many projects were pilots, funded and operated for a specific period, and were frequently isolated or on the periphery of health services, rather than being integral to core business. Projects were often initiated by innovative sponsors, and allowed to languish if the sponsor moved on. Where applications were formally adopted on a long-term basis, they often remained within specific environments rather than being implemented throughout the agency. Limited infrastructure, a lack of data standards, legal and ethical issues, and user resistance all prevented many projects from becoming integrated into mainstream services. Even today, many programs continue to remain on the periphery, with little attention given to making systematic organisational changes to support their sustainability. 'One of the key findings from the study in 2000 is that currently in the **e-health** sector in Australia, spending in IT is much greater at the non-solutions, ad-hoc projects level rather than at the total solutions/strategic spending level' (McGill 2001, p. 2).

These discrete projects represent a typical approach to an emerging field or practice. Such an approach enables us to build our knowledge about health information systems, while not committing too heavily to unproven technology or systems. Unfortunately, this limits the ability of successful projects to make a broader impact on the overall effectiveness and efficiency of health services. Consider the following:

- In-house administrative and clinical information systems may enable timely access to health information within a single enterprise, but they do not reduce the demand for services. In fact, as the population ages, and as diseases of affluence increase, we can expect demands for services to increase.
- Discrete enterprise-based systems do not facilitate efficient access to health information as individual consumers move around and across services.
- Ad hoc projects do not facilitate the collection of information to enable identification of longer term trends and effective planning of health care services.

Strategic directions

In recent years, governments and service providers have become aware of the need for a more strategic, integrated approach to information management. We see this in a shift from the discrete, stand-alone projects to a focus on regional, state-wide, and nation-wide models of information management. We also see it in efforts to develop infrastructure, protocols, and standards; in the focus on encouraging new partnerships and relationships between organisations, health professionals, and consumers; and in encouragement to these organisations to collaborate and share information. Box 1.9 illustrates the move towards strategic thinking.

BOX 1.9

STRATEGIC APPROACHES TO INFORMATION MANAGEMENT

Australia

The Australian Government will provide $128.3 million over the next four years towards the implementation of a national health information network, called Health*Connect*, as a major platform for reforming health care delivery in Australia...**HealthConnect**... involves the electronic collection, storage and exchange of consumer health information via a secure network and within strict **privacy** safeguards (Commonwealth Department of Health and Ageing 2004).

Canada

There are a number of key priorities to be addressed in the development of a health infrastructure in Canada. Stakeholders across the country, including the HIHD, are addressing such topics as: electronic health records, integrated provider solutions, protection of personal health information, standards, telehealth, and change management (Health Canada E-health Resource Centre 2004).

New Zealand

The New Zealand government focus is to invest in, and promote, key items of health information management infrastructure, particularly in the primary health care sector. The infrastructure includes the National Health Index, the Medical Warning System, a national clinical coding system for primary health care as well as for hospitals, the early adoption of a standard for health messaging, and a national health intranet and the appropriate security apparatus (New Zealand Ministry of Health 2004b).

United Kingdom

Over the last decade, the UK's health policy has increasingly considered the role of information and information technologies in the provision of health care. More recently, in policy terms, that role has changed and expanded and includes not only administrative and managerial support but also assisting frontline staff in delivering benefits to patients and bringing new services to communities and into individual homes (Cornford et al. 2003).

USA

Use of modern information technology has the potential to transform the delivery of health care in America for the better...The federal government will provide a vision and a strategic direction for a national interoperable health care system...(US Department of Health and Human Services 2004).

These efforts are expected to produce more strategic outcomes, including the following:

- Generation of data and information. This will enable public health professionals to identify longer term trends and implement effective planning of health care services.
- More effective and efficient use of limited health care resources. Information and communication technologies will enable clinicians and patients to develop new ways of accessing information and communicating with one another.
- Promotion of evidence-based practice as health professionals access online medical databases and other information sources for the latest research results and information to inform their decisions. Hand-held devices, personal computers, and terminals in the wards will provide access to both patient information and expert advice at the point of care.
- Coordination and monitoring of care for individual patients as administrative and clinical information systems integrate and disseminate data and information from diverse sources. This will make it possible to maintain patient files as consumers move within and between services.
- Informed and empowered consumers accessing information from a variety of sources. This will enable them to be actively involved in their own health care.

While these outcomes are expected to enhance health care, there is a growing argument that they will not be sufficient to resolve the problems, and that we need to take a radically different approach. 'Given that commentators today are alarmed at the current strains on the health system, we have to assume that by 2020 the health care systems in most nations will either have somehow transformed substantially or will have failed...it may require nothing less than the reinvention of health care' (Coiera 2004, p. 1197).

Reinventing health care

One of the characteristics of being in the old world (or paradigm) is that it's almost impossible to imagine the new one (Smith 2004a, p. 328).

There are different ideas about how a reinvented health care system will look and operate. Berwick (2002, p. 2) envisions a system that offers ' "24/7/365" access to help that is uncompromising, meeting whatever need exists, whenever and wherever it exists, in whatever form requested.' While this is more than most think possible, or perhaps even desirable, there is consensus that information is the key and that the increasing use of technological and other information and communications systems to access this information will fundamentally change the roles of consumers and health professionals and the way health care services are structured and accessed.

Reinventing the consumer as partner

> The first development is that patients have access to the same information, knowledge and guidelines as clinicians...sometimes people will manage their own problems (Smith 2004a, p. 328).

The move towards community-based care, health promotion, and active consumer involvement offers the opportunity for the transfer of knowledge from professionals to the wider community, offering the opportunity for a significant break from the established approach to health care. This can be facilitated by creating information systems that enable consumer access to the most reliable and current health and medical information. While some specialist knowledge will always remain the province of specific health professional groups, there is much that could be available to health consumers.

Some might view increased consumer control as dangerous, arguing that consumers may not understand the information they access, may not know when they should consult a health professional, and that they need guidance. This may be true. On the other hand, reports of patients coming to harm as the result of online advice are rare, whereas accounts of those who have obtained better care, averted medical mistakes, or saved their own lives are common (Ferguson & Frydman 2004, p. 1147). And many consumers are comfortable with the concept of self-management. 'Many e-patients say that the medical information and guidance they can find online is more complete and useful than what they receive from their clinicians' (Ferguson & Frydman 2004, p. 1148). There is a concern, however, as Box 1.10 indicates, that the quality of online information varies and if health services adopt the consumer-as-partner approach, they may need to play a role in ensuring that consumers are able to evaluate the quality of information they find.

Reinventing health care does not mean abandoning consumers. It means viewing them as equal partners capable of making decisions and managing much of their own health and medical care. It is already happening in the management of chronic diseases, where the concept of *Expert Patients* is increasingly discussed. 'Expert Patients Programmes are not simply about educating or instructing patients about their condition and then measuring success on the basis of patient compliance. They are based on developing the confidence and motivation of patients to use their own skills and knowledge to take effective control' (UK Department of Health 2001, p. 6).

Reinventing access to services

The face-to-face consultation was once the primary source of information gathering and sharing. This function has declined as diagnostic technology is used increasingly for gathering medical information. Yet the face-to-face consultation continues to be a significant element of contemporary health care delivery, consuming a considerable

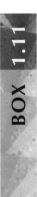

QUALITY OF HEALTH INFORMATION ON THE INTERNET

There were several examples of good quality and well-presented information within sites that had been carefully constructed and kept up to date...There were few examples of misleading and biased information but many more examples of information 'gaps' and a concentration on relatively minor details (Bouchier & Bath 2003, p. 17).

A report by Stone et al. (2002), supported by the Commonwealth Fund found that while a growing number of consumers are turning to the Internet for information on health and health care, much of what they are finding on websites—especially about physicians—is unreliable. According to the report, 'only 25 of the 40 sites examined (63 per cent) posted doctors' medical school, while just 10 (25 per cent) listed their number of years in practice' (p. 3).

percentage of our health resources. There is increasing support for the view that this could, or should change, and that we need to create alternative pathways for accessing the health care system (Berwick 2002, Smith 2004, Yellowlees 2000). This does not mean abandoning the face-to-face consultation. It does mean that we need to provide alternatives where a face-to-face consultation is not needed. These might include online consultations, group visits, email consultations, or even chat rooms. 'The access we need to create is access to help and healing, and that does not always mean—in fact I think it rarely means—reliance on face-to-face meetings between patients, doctors, and nurses' (Berwick 2002, p. 42).

REINVENTING ACCESS TO SERVICES

Patients will have access to the same information, knowledge, and guidelines as clinicians. Access to professional services will be via the Web. Patients will enter data online and be advised that care is not needed, be referred to patients' organisations, or be passed directly to a clinician. The clinician may not be a doctor, but may be a nurse or other health care worker supported by technology that will provide instant access to knowledge and management pathways. Doctors will be supported by technology that will guide their management of patients. Many consultations will happen via the Internet (Smith 2004a).

Tempering expectations

Once more we have high expectations for health informatics. Today, however, these expectations are tempered by our understanding that we need to do more than simply introduce these systems into the health care environment. We understand that the introduction of information management systems will challenge many of the assumptions and structures underpinning the traditional health care environment. Information and communications systems are designed for collaboration and information sharing. They may require health professionals to interact with one another in ways not previously explored. In addition, health information systems often disrupt traditional **work routines**, workflow and work relationships. The location of equipment, the need to consult with others, the protocols involved and the need to enter and access information in a timely manner may all have an impact on workflow and routines. This may or may not be perceived as a good thing.

With the benefit of past experience, we understand that if we are to meet expectations, information management systems must be designed to take into account the complexity of the health care environment and the needs, priorities, and agendas of key players.

SUMMARY

During the latter half of the twentieth century there was a strong expectation that health informatics and its associated technologies would contribute to improved health care. This optimism reflected the belief in science and technology that has shaped our modern worldview.

In biomedicine—the application of the scientific worldview to health care—this belief in science appears to have been well founded. Biomedicine is widely accepted as contributing to improved health outcomes in many Western countries. In the last hundred years we have seen a decrease in infectious diseases, formerly untreatable conditions being successfully managed, and life expectancy has increased for many groups. Advances in biomedicine, however, have also resulted in increased demands for services, increased complex interventions, and rapidly rising health care costs.

The success of biomedicine has also resulted in an ever-expanding knowledge base. In seeking to manage this knowledge and its application, the health care environment has evolved into a complex hierarchy of specialties and subspecialties. Health care services are organised around these specialties and across public and private sector organisations. As a consequence, episodes of treatment may involve multiple health professionals and organisations. This results in the generation of increasing amounts of health information, which together with biomedical knowledge informs the decision-making process of health professionals. The complexity of the health care environment means that the management and communication of this information and knowledge is becoming problematic. In recent years, the emphasis on consumer-centred service delivery, continuity of care across services, evidence-based practice, and a move of resources and services beyond traditional hospital-based care into community care and preventative programs has contributed to this problem

This need to manage biomedical knowledge and health information more effectively and efficiently gave rise to the discipline of health informatics. Although the early optimism about the discipline was not realised, hindsight suggests that this was due, at least in part, to the technocentric focus of early work, which did not adequately consider the cultural and organisational health care environment within which health informatics operates. We now appreciate that if health informatics is to live up to expectations, we need to understand both the tools and techniques of information management, and the complexity of the health care environment.

Adopting this perspective is broadening our thinking about the potential of health informatics, taking us beyond the view that information systems will slot neatly into the existing health care environment. Today we realise that health informatics has the potential to support dramatic and widespread changes to the structures and operations of health care. There is a growing view that this is not only possible, but also essential if our health care services are to fulfil their role.

These ideas are reflected in the perception of health informatics as a unique discipline: 'The health care environment is markedly different from business and therefore demands an identifiable discipline, health informatics. A discipline based on socio-technical approaches' (Atkinson et al. 2001, p. 1).

WWW LINKS

These websites offer more detail about several issues raised in this chapter. They represent the tip of the iceberg. It is recommended that you exercise your skills in seeking out and evaluating information on the Internet.

Evaluating web resources

Beck, S. 2004, 'The good, the bad and the ugly, or, why it's a good idea to evaluate Web resources' <http://lib.nmsu.edu/instruction/eval.html>

Health systems

Liu, E. & Lee, V. 1998, 'Health care expenditure and financing in Australia, accessing physician information on the Internet' <http://www.legco.gov.hk/yr97-98/english/sec/library/11plc.pdf>

Changing roles and relationships

Gillespie, R., 2002, 'Changing relationships: findings from the Patient Involvement Project', Executive Summary, King's Fund, United Kingdom <http://www.kingsfund.org.uk/pdf/ChangingRelationshipsSummary.pdf>

Trends in health information management

HealthOnline: A Health Information Action Plan for Australia <http://www.ahic.org.au/downloads/actplan2.pdf>

Health Canada: Information, Analysis and Connectivity Branch <http://www.hc-sc.gc.ca/iacb-dgiac/english/>

New Zealand Health Strategy, online version <http://www.maorihealt.govt.nz/download.php?id=NZHthStrat.pdf>

CRITICAL THINKING

Roberta is a young athlete. She has come to see Dr Geepee for two reasons. First, she has developed a skin rash from shaving her legs. Dr Geepee writes a prescription for an antibiotic. Roberta also has a problem with extreme fatigue following training or competing. After discussing her training program, diet, and symptoms, Dr Geepee suggests that she may have an iron-deficiency problem. Checking this will require a blood test from the local pathology laboratory, and treatment would involve consultations with a sports nutritionist. The Institute of Sport is conducting a research project into the main health problems experienced by young female athletes and is seeking data from Dr Geepee. The research will assist the national athletics body to develop policies relating to appropriate training and dietary regimes for young women athletes.

1 Trace Roberta's progress through the system. Identify points where she interacts with health professionals and administrators, where health professionals might communicate and where health data and information might be shared.

2 Identify points in Roberta's experiences where information systems might impact on service choices, professional relationships, patient–professional relationships, and administrative aspects of service delivery.

3 What cultural, political and/or economic factors might impact on the introduction of health information systems at the points identified?

4 If Roberta were accessing another of the five health systems discussed in this chapter, what differences would there be for choice of services (ability to choose professionals, public/private, and so on), health insurance, and payment options.

5 Use the ideas from Box 1.11 to redesign Roberta's interaction with the health system. What issues can you identify with implementing this model?

CHAPTER 2

WHAT IS HEALTH INFORMATICS?

OVERVIEW

Health informatics is defined as an evolving socio-technical and scientific discipline. Its subject matter is the collection, storage, retrieval, communication, and optimal use of health-related data, information, and knowledge. The socio-technical perspective shapes the specific issues explored within the subject matter, while the adoption of scientific method shapes the methodology used to explore these issues. Yet health informatics is a complex field involving many different disciplines and groups, each with their own view on priorities, issues, and solutions. This has implications for the development of the discipline and the **profession.**

OBJECTIVES

At the completion of this chapter, you should have an understanding of:
- the focus of health informatics
- the issues explored by the discipline
- the issues faced by the discipline
- the issues faced by the profession
- the perspectives of key players shaping the discipline and the profession.

CONCEPTS

Informatics	**Positivist research**
Health informatics	Critical research
Profession	Qualitative
Theory	Quantitative
Interpretive research	

INTRODUCTION

This chapter explores the discipline of health informatics. It begins by defining the broader concept of informatics before identifying factors in the health care environment that gave rise to a distinct discipline. The discussion then focuses on health informatics, examining elements of the definition and exploring the scope and focus of the discipline. The relationship between the discipline and the profession is also considered. The chapter concludes by identifying a number of key player perspectives and exploring the implications of these different perspectives for the application of the discipline in the health care environment.

INFORMATICS

Think information, not computers (Newbold 2002, p. 20).

Many people think informatics is about computers. Since the emergence of informatics was linked with the uptake of computers in business and commerce, this is understandable, if not quite accurate.

Until the end of the Second World War computers were the province of the military and scientific fraternity. During the 1950s and 1960s computers emerged in government, industrial, and commercial environments. They were initially introduced to facilitate data storage and data processing.

The science of information management also emerged in the 1960s. The French *informatique*, the Russian *informatik* and the English *informatics* were terms coined to describe this emerging science. The juxtaposition of these two events resulted in the perception that **informatics** was primarily about the use of computers to process information. Yet individuals and organisations also process information. The emerging discipline acknowledged this, and from the beginning informatics focused on the 'representation, processing and communication of information in natural and artificial systems' (Fourman 2002, p. 1). Computing and communication technology are the tools used to facilitate information management. 'We often use computers in information management, but they are our tools, just as stethoscopes or catheters might be yours. The true focus of informatics is on handling information' (Abbott 2002, p. 14).

This is an important point because the focus of the discipline will shape the issues it identifies and the questions it asks. A technology focus might ask, 'What is the best technology for achieving the desired outcome?' This precludes the possibility of non-technical solutions. An information management focus, on the other hand, might ask:

- What information is needed?
- By whom?
- Where and when?
- What is the best means of providing this information?

The answers to these questions may point to a non-technical solution. As Coiera observes, 'it is possible for a well-designed set of paper forms to be far more effective than poorly designed computer-based ones' (1997, p. 64). This highlights the point that if we ask the wrong questions, we may never consider the best solutions.

Information and communications technology are, however, the primary tools of information management and must necessarily feature, if not star, in discussions on the subject.

HEALTH INFORMATICS: A SPECIAL CASE?

The health care environment is markedly different from business and therefore demands an identifiable discipline, 'health informatics' (Atkinson et al. 2001, p. 1).

From the early 1960s, computers were being used to process information in health organisations. These early applications were largely used for the business aspects of health care. 'The rapidly expanding health care industry began using computers to track patient charges, calculate payrolls, control inventory and analyse medical statistics' (Hannah et al. 1999, p. 28). These systems were primarily data processing systems and the nature, scope, and development of computer technology at the time supported these uses rather than more sophisticated data analysis and **knowledge management** systems. Administrative applications were also the focus in other industries and the transfer to the health care environment was an obvious development. While there was some interest in using computers for the management of clinical information, the limitations of the technology and the complexities of biomedical knowledge meant that the potential for clinical applications was obvious to only a few pioneers. Interest in the use of computers to manage medical, nursing, and other clinical information grew throughout the 1970s and it was the increasing efforts to use informatics in the clinical domain that brought about the realisation that a specialised discipline might be required. Factors pointing to the need for a specialised discipline included:

- the nature of biomedical information
- the complexity of the health care environment.

The nature of biomedical information

Information retrieval

It is an inherent requirement of modern health care that the most current biomedical knowledge is available to practitioners. Yet the ever-increasing size of the knowledge base means that keeping up with new information is a constant challenge for health professionals. The potential for computers to assist with meeting this challenge was apparent even before a **health informatics** discipline emerged. Biomedical information lent itself readily to the electronic filing, dissemination, and retrieval functions characteristic of early computer systems. The US National Library of Medicine began to develop **MEDLARS**, a computerised literature-retrieval system, during the 1960s.

Since that time, the challenge to disseminate the most up-to-date research and other medical information has been an ongoing issue for health informatics. The emphasis on evidence-based practice ensures that it remains a central issue for clinicians, while the increasing trend for patients to take more responsibility for their own health and well-being means that it is increasingly an issue for patients. Box 2.1 lists some information retrieval systems currently in use.

BOX 2.1

FACILITATING INFORMATION RETRIEVAL FOR CLINICIANS AND PATIENTS

MedlinePlus is a free online information service offered by the US National Library of Medicine and the National Institutes of Health. It includes information about medical diseases, and prescription and non-prescription drugs, plus lists of hospitals and physicians, a medical encyclopaedia, a medical dictionary, and links to clinical trials.

The Cochrane Collaboration is an international non-profit organisation that began as a small group of clinicians who identified the need for an evidence basis to published research material. It produces systematic reviews of research materials, clinical trials and other studies of interventions.

BMJ.com is a site that commenced in May 1995 and includes the full text of all articles published in the weekly *British Medical Journal* since January 1994. It also contains some material that is unique to the website.

HealthInsite is an Australian Government initiative, funded by the Commonwealth Department of Health and Ageing and is directed towards health consumers. It seeks to provide online access to information about a range of medical conditions, health matters, and lifestyle issues.

The clinical domain

> The goal of automating diagnosis was perhaps one of the earliest goals of medical informatics, dating back to the early 1960s (Altman 1997, p. 118).

Although there was an early interest in using computers to manage clinical information, biomedical knowledge did not lend itself quite so readily to the sophisticated computer manipulations required for clinical analysis and decision support. This was due, at least in part, to the nature of biomedical knowledge. Data typically dealt with in business, commerce, and health administration computing systems tends to be fairly uniform, and is relatively easily structured for use in information technology. Biomedical knowledge is often difficult to explain or communicate, and is not as easily structured, organised, or manipulated. This is because biomedical knowledge is 'fuzzy'. **Fuzzy knowledge** is imprecise, and interpretation is often a matter of degree. Box 2.2 illustrates the fuzzy nature of biomedical knowledge.

Thus, while biomedical knowledge is assumed to be empirical, objective, and factual it is also incomplete. Each patient brings a unique combination of symptoms, personal circumstances, and expectations to a consultation. We have yet to create a doctor-in-a-box capable of demonstrating the intuition, knowledge, wisdom, and judgment needed for this type of clinical decision-making.

The challenge of dealing with fuzzy medical knowledge has been a significant area of interest since the discipline of health informatics first emerged. It has given rise to at least two particular areas of endeavour:

- *Decision support and expert systems*: Medical informatics has led the way in expert systems. One of the first expert systems, called **MYCIN**, was developed in 1975 to diagnose and recommend therapy for blood diseases.

BOX 2.2

DIAGNOSING AND RECORDING FUZZY KNOWLEDGE

Diagnosis: In a clinical situation the patient may complain of headache, shivering, abdominal pain, and vomiting. These are all symptoms that, according to the relative importance of each, will lead the clinician towards one diagnosis or another. For example, all of these symptoms are compatible with influenza, which in many countries would be the commonest cause and most likely diagnosis. In children these symptoms can also point strongly towards pneumonia involving the lower lobe of the right lung, and in others a diagnosis of acute appendicitis could be considered. Many other conditions could, under certain circumstances, come into consideration. These include meningitis, malaria, diverticulitis, cerebral abscess, tonsillitis, infectious mononucleosis (glandular fever), and more. To make a diagnosis, the clinician must draw on biomedical knowledge, but also on his or her own expertise, and knowledge of the individual patient. Clinicians use this fuzzy logic in most clinical situations.

Recording: Health professionals make observations and notes using unstructured natural language. As a consequence, despite use of specific medical terminology, many concepts remain somewhat loose and open to interpretation. Take, for example, a reactive cardiotocograph reading—a printout of a baby's heart tracing. Many health care practitioners may describe a CTG reading as reactive. This description does not provide information about frequency and intensity, or indicate whether the health practitioner is reassured or concerned by the reading. The term *reactive* is open to interpretation by other health professionals. While these types of terms are frequently used in health records, their exact interpretation may vary widely.

- *Standards and terminology*: Before medical and health knowledge can be shared electronically, standards that will enable it to be communicated and interpreted must be developed. The development of controlled **vocabularies**, taxonomies, and classification systems has been, and continues to be, an important area of health/medical informatics.

The health care environment

> The particular social, professional and cultural context of health care is a major factor that dominates health informatics (Altman 1997, p. 119).

The nature of the health environment also contributed to the emergence of health informatics. Chapter 1 represented contemporary health systems as typically:

- large and complex
- a mix of public and private providers in community and hospital settings
- a mix of clinical and other professions
- characterised by multiple lines of authority and responsibility
- subject to issues of power, agendas, and priorities, which affect relationships between professional groups and organisations.

Patients typically move within and between departments and services. Clinical and administrative data and information also move within and across departmental and service boundaries. The bulk of this information is of a private and confidential nature, and its collection, storage, and use are subject to legal and ethical guidelines.

While informatics applications focused on administrative systems for individual departments and organisations, the complexity of the health environment was not identified as an issue. By the 1970s, however, with increasing interest in clinical information systems and the consequent need for information flow across departments and organisations, the complex social and organisational characteristics of the health environment began to create challenges not found in most business and commercial environments. Issues for health informatics include:

- *Privacy and security*: The extremely sensitive nature of health data and information requires that privacy and confidentiality be stringently protected. At the same time, appropriate information needs to be available for use by properly authorised people. Privacy and security issues become more pressing and more complex as information increasingly flows across departments and organisations. The complex mix of users and technical standards found in the health care environment make privacy and security significant challenges.
- *Integrating technology into clinical workflows*: Issues include not only minimising disruption to routines but also dealing with the possible impact of technology on roles and relationships. These changes are not always welcome.
- *Usability*: ensuring that applications are easy to learn and to use. **Usability** is considered to be a very significant factor in the acceptance of information systems by health professionals.

- *Identifying the optimum information tools for each clinical setting*: Clinical environments vary widely and some tools, even when they are performing the same functions, are more suited to some environments than others.

The discipline emerges

As informatics professionals and health professionals grappled with the unique characteristics of the health care environment, an identifiable discipline began to emerge. From the early 1970s national and international organisations were being formed to explore issues around the management of health information. As these issues were identified, the parameters of the field began to be defined. Box 2.3 lists some milestones in this process. For a more detailed account of the development of the discipline, see the readings at the end of the chapter.

BOX 2.3

MILESTONES IN THE EMERGENCE OF THE DISCIPLINE

1980   Dr Morris Collen defined medical informatics.
1983   Dr Marion Ball coined the phrase *nursing informatics*.
1989   Dr Salah Mandil coined the phrase *health informatics*.
1989   The International Medical Informatics Association (IMIA), formerly the Fourth Technical Committee of the International Federation for Information Processing, became an international organisation in its own right.

HEALTH INFORMATICS IS AN EVOLVING DISCIPLINE

Health informatics is evolving from an area of interest to a discipline in its own right. Musen and van Bemmel encapsulate this evolution: 'During the past three or four decades, we have transitioned from a group of hospital-based technologists whose primary focus was the implementation of clinical information systems to a diverse community of scholars, clinicians, engineers and pragmatists' (2003, p. 209). There are two dimensions to this evolution, involving a move from:

- a technocentric perspective to a socio-technical perspective
- an interest in medical systems to an interest in health systems.

Technocentric to socio-technical

To design sociotechnical systems, we must understand how people and technologies interact (Coiera 2004, p. 1197).

Health informatics, or medical informatics, as it was first called, emerged as a special interest area for computing professionals and computer-minded medical professionals. These origins are reflected in Collen's 1980 definition of the field as the 'application of computers to all fields of medicine—medical care, medical education and medical research' (in Tolentino 1999, p. 1), and there was great interest in what the technology could or should do in the clinical environment. Implicit in this focus was the scientific worldview of technology as progress or, to use Coiera's phrase (2004, p. 1197), 'technology as king'. This view shaped discussion, policies and research programs for much of the 1970s and 1980s and on into the 1990s.

As the discipline evolved, the limitations of a technology focus became apparent. Many early projects were less successful than was expected and research pointed to the need to understand political, cultural, and organisational issues. Medical informatics began to draw on other disciplines, particularly the social sciences of information systems, sociology, and social psychology. This modified the technocentric focus, and by the end of the 1990s, health informatics was increasingly viewed as 'an evolving socio-technical and scientific discipline that deals with the collection, storage, retrieval, communication and optimal use of health related data, information and knowledge' (HISA 2004).

The adoption of a multi-disciplinary, socio-technical perspective enabled the discipline to explore issues arising from the interaction between information systems and the social, professional, and cultural contexts of health care. This includes issues of power and influence, professional agendas and priorities at the organisational, departmental and individual level. It also includes issues around roles and relationships, work routines, and procedures, change management and **innovation diffusion**, education, and professional development. Table 2.1 illustrates this multi-disciplinary influence.

While interaction between people, technology, and the workplace is now firmly on the agenda, the technocentric focus continues to have an influence. Coiera goes so far as to suggest that:

> The sacred ground of health informatics remains anything to do with computers, the web, information architectures, the electronic health record, and heroic challenges such as the creation of enormous terminology systems. The profane ground of health informatics, still mostly shunned, is the world of politics, culture and persuasion, complaints from users when systems disappoint them, the messy craft of system implementation, which requires different tactics from one site to the next, and our unacceptably high number of system failures (2004, p. 1197).

Medical to health informatics

As the discipline evolved from a technocentric to a socio-technical perspective, the focus also broadened from medical care, education, and research to a more comprehensive coverage of the health environment. As this move progressed, the term 'medical' was considered unable to convey adequately the broadening focus. The term 'health informatics' began to be used to describe the range of activities, interests, and players—both medical and non-medical— within the health care field, while terms such as medical informatics and nursing informatics were increasingly applied to narrower areas of activity.

Table 2.1 Multi-disciplinary influence on health informatics

Discipline	Questions
Informatics	What is information?
Sociology	What human and societal values support health? Health sociology information technologies? What is the impact of technology on various groups within health care and society? Are health informatics applications desirable?
Psychology	How do the characteristics of end-users affect the design of health information systems? What cognitive constraints should be taken into account in the deployment of information systems? What technologies better support people's decisions?
Social psychology	How do organisations affect the generation, flow, and use of information systems information? What type of social organisation supports informatics applications? How do different types of users interact with information technology? What role do economic factors play in the uptake of information? What is the role of information technology in organisational change? How is the social organisation of information technologies influenced by social forces and social practices?
Computer science	What are the preferred networking solutions? What algorithms are required to accomplish specific tasks? What is the role of AI systems (expert systems, decision support systems, and rule-based and perception-based systems)? How do we ensure security?

Source: created from: Arocha, 2003

Yet, while 'health informatics' is increasingly used as the term to convey the broader focus of informatics in health care, the term 'medical informatics' continues to be used. This is due in part to regional differences. In Europe, '"medical" tends to include the full range of health professions, while in other places, most notably the United States, "medical" generally refers to physicians only' (MacDougall & Brittain 1994). It is also territorial. 'The difference between "health informatics" and "medical informatics" reflects largely territorial (political) difference between disciplines. Both camps claim to have a multi- or interdisciplinary approach' (McKenzie 2000, p. 1). This highlights the political nature of both the health care environment and health informatics.

Within the broad discipline of health informatics a number of sub-disciplines have evolved. These include:

- medical informatics
- nursing informatics

- public health informatics
- bioinformatics
- consumer health informatics.

Medical informatics

> For the moment, a distinction will remain between health informaticians and medical informaticians—these are clinicians...who apply medical (doctor) skills and responsibilities to their work (Hayes 2002 in Taylor 2002, p. 3).

Medical informatics professionals argue that while they share the general focus of other health informatics subsets, medical informatics has developed its own areas of interest and approaches that set it apart. They argue that the medical informatics professional requires specific medical/clinical knowledge in addition to information management and information technology skills and knowledge.

Nursing informatics

Nursing informatics was recognised in 1992 by the American Nurses Association as a separate area of study within the overall discipline of health informatics. As a subset of health informatics, nursing informatics professionals acknowledge that they have much in common with other health informatics professionals. However, the particular focus of nursing informatics is on the discipline of *nursing* and the use of data, information, and knowledge to support nursing practice, education, and research.

Public health informatics

Public health informatics is the application of health information systems and strategies to public health research, education and practice. The focus of public health informatics is not on the treatment of individuals, but on the health status of groups and communities. Rather than collecting data for specific individuals, public health informatics collects and analyses large amounts of aggregated, depersonalised data and information. This includes data about healthy individuals and those suffering different diseases or conditions.

Bioinformatics

Bioinformatics is concerned with the collection, organisation, and analysis of complex biological structures, specifically the genome sciences. It has emerged as a result of advances in both informatics and biology. A major focus of bioinformatics is the development of databases and algorithms to enable biological research, particularly genomic research.

Consumer health informatics

Consumer health informatics focuses on identifying consumer information needs and developing systems and strategies to enable consumers to access that information. Despite the emergence of consumer groups, it is not uncommon for consumer informatics to be mediated by health professionals, administrators, and/or government. Where this is the case, there tends to be an emphasis on educating consumers to access valid, high quality information, and limited exploration of issues around the consumer as an equal partner in all levels of health from policy development to individual care.

Health informatics is a scientific discipline

> The scientific underpinnings of the field are not well articulated in our textbooks or by our professional societies (Musen & van Bemmel 2002, p. 195).

Since the nineteenth and twentieth centuries were dominated by the rational scientific worldview, many emerging fields of endeavour sought legitimacy by defining themselves as scientific disciplines. Health informatics is one of these.

The scientific worldview stressed the objective, ordered nature of the world and advocated scientific method as the means of identifying and understanding this structure. A scientific discipline uses scientific method for developing and structuring the knowledge of the field. Scientific method, first applied in the physical sciences, produces knowledge by developing theories and then testing those theories through research—the collection of data or empirical evidence.

Health informatics and theory

> Many investigators within the medical informatics community are perceived to have difficulty articulating the underlying theories and principles that guide their work (Musen & van Bemmel 2002, p. 195).

Theories are the foundation of a discipline. They are used to explain:

- what the physical or social world is like
- how that world changes
- why it changes.

A **theory** begins with observations about physical or social phenomena. Repeated observations of the same phenomena lead to the questions what, how, and why? This results in the formulation of a **hypothesis**, which is a tentative explanation for the phenomena. The hypothesis forms the basis of research, the results of which lead to the acceptance or rejection of the hypothesis. If the hypothesis is supported, it may then become a new theory and thus contribute to the knowledge base of the discipline. A theory remains valid while evidence continues to support it and no evidence appears to refute it. Thus, the knowledge base expands and changes.

Each discipline develops theories to build its own specific area of knowledge. The emerging discipline of health informatics has focused on solving the practical problems in the health care environment. In doing so, it has drawn on its multi-disciplinary base, rather than develop its own theories. Theories used by health informatics include:

- **systems theory**
- organisational theory and models

- organisation development and change theories
- learning theories.

Drawing on a range of disciplines for theoretical input helps ensure the relevance of health informatics to the many different environments and professions in health care. At the same time, this has resulted in health informatics not yet having its own underlying theory to set it apart as a distinct discipline. This is a concern for some: 'We need to define our paradigm and to demonstrate how our research collectively builds on a common theory. Of course, articulating that theory remains a major academic challenge for us' (Musen & van Bemmel 2002, p. 195).

Health informatics research

The scientific method was originally a tool of the physical sciences, which deal with inanimate objects in the physical world. The social sciences, including health informatics, explore human attributes such as attitudes, opinions, and emotions, and abstract concepts such as power and authority. These phenomena cannot be adequately studied using only the approaches and methods applied to inanimate objects. Therefore health informatics, as with other social sciences, draws upon several methods for its scientific research (Neuman 2000, pp. 63–81). These are:

- *Positivist research*: Also known as positivism, this approach most closely follows that of the physical sciences.
- *Interpretive research*: This method emphasises the need to understand the social world from the perspective of the participants.
- *Critical research*: This approach focuses on questioning the established social structures and relationships.

Research involves the collection and analysis of data according to clearly defined rules, procedures, and techniques (methods). Data may be either quantitative (expressed numerically), or qualitative (expressed as words, images, or objects). Positivist research has traditionally emphasised quantitative data, interpretive research has emphasised qualitative methods, and critical research uses both. While both quantitative and qualitative methods are accepted in the social sciences, supporters of each method are often critical of the other (Neuman 2000, p. 16). Yet, as Table 2.2 demonstrates, the different approaches need not be mutually exclusive or in competition with each other. They can be complementary.

The approach and related method depends on the context, subject matter, and purpose of the research. Today, a combination of methods is frequently adopted. Software usability, for example, is assessed in terms of how quickly and accurately tasks can be completed (positivist), and of how much users like using the software (interpretive). It has been suggested, however, that research in health informatics has tended to be predominantly qualitative, rather than quantitative, and this is viewed as a weakness of the discipline (Bowns et al. 1999, Coiera 2003).

Table 2.2 Research questions and methods

Clinical field	Empirical research question	Quantitative research method for that question	Interpretive research question	Qualitative research method for that question
Lung cancer	Do the vitamin supplements alpha-tocopherol and beta-carotene prevent lung and other cancers in male smokers in Finland?	Randomised controlled trial	What is the impact of specialist palliative care on the quality of life for patients suffering lung cancer?	Individual (semi-structured) interviews Focus groups Cross-validation between different interviewers
Cystic fibrosis	What is the effect of different doses of tauroursodeoxy-cholic acid on children suffering cystic fibrosis?	Double-blind crossover randomised control study	What is the experience of mothers caring for a child with cystic fibrosis?	Individual (semi-structured) interviews Respondent validation
Chronic fatigue syndrome	What is the efficacy of an educational intervention explaining symptoms to encourage graded exercise in patients with chronic fatigue syndrome?	Randomised control trial	How does educational intervention impact on the way patients with chronic fatigue syndrome participate and experience graded exercise?	Individual (semi-structured) interviews Focus group discussions Respondent validation

Health informatics is information management

[Information management is] assuring that the right information is available to the right people, within and without an organisation, at the right time and place and for the right price (Wright 2002).

Musen and van Bemmel state that 'our research community is dedicated to the study of information' (2003, p. 210). Consequently, information management is at the very heart of health informatics. Health professionals, whether caring for an individual patient, making decisions at an organisational level, or seeking information about a whole population, are dependent on accurate data and information. It is essential that this data and information is collected, stored, retrieved, and communicated as effectively and efficiently as possible. This raises a number of ongoing issues for health informatics, including:

- *Privacy*: Health and medical data is one of the most sensitive forms of data and information gathered about individuals. Maintaining confidentiality to the level desired is a problem for all information systems that manage personal health information.
- *Professional*: There are a number of issues around access to, and sharing of professional information.
- *Legal*: Confidentiality, unauthorised use, and liability are significant issues in relation to electronic communication and consultation.
- *Standards*: The incompatibility of many existing systems is a consequence of the lack of common standards for health care technologies. This is one of the major barriers to the increased integration of databases and other systems.
- *Security*: The increasingly integrated information management environment has created significant issues around information protection.
- *Technical*: Problems arise around data types—clinical data comes in a combination of text, codes, speech, and images.

AND HEALTH INFORMATICS PROFESSIONALS...

Health informatics is having a mid-life crisis, it is a 45 year old profession wandering around the desert to find itself (Shahar 2001).

While a discipline is not at all the same as a profession, the two are nevertheless linked. A profession is an occupation requiring specialised education for a clearly defined area of employment. Characteristics of a profession include:

- the possession of expert knowledge not possessed by the layperson
- certification or accreditation of educational qualifications
- governance over one's professional field—for example, setting entrance requirements and handling discipline of one's colleagues. This generally includes the development of a code of ethics.

Health informatics is moving towards attaining professional status. National organisations and associations, in conjunction with international organisations such as the International Medical Informatics Association (IMIA), are developing guidelines, standards, and codes of ethics for the health informatics professional and there are moves to establish registration and governance. Organisations and their membership reflect the fluid boundaries of the discipline. As Box 2.4 shows, membership of associations is very broad, and recognition of qualifications is a moving feast.

While the move towards creating a professional niche is relatively recent, information management has long had a role in health care, and many existing information management roles are being absorbed into the emerging health informatics profession. Box 2.5 gives an indication of some of the roles/job titles currently falling within the area. These job titles are by no means definitive. Different titles are used in different health systems. Box 2.6 shows the spread of the profession across the health care environment.

BOX 2.4

ORGANISATIONS, MEMBERSHIP, GOALS

International
The International Medical Informatics Association (IMIA) seeks to promote informatics in health care and biomedical research. Members are both individuals involved or interested in health informatics and organisations involved in the field. IMIA has developed a Code of Ethics for Health Information Professionals, which seeks to provide ethical guidance and shape professional behaviour.

Australia
The Health Informatics Society of Australia (HISA) seeks to improve health care through health informatics. This includes provision of education curriculum development, teaching and training, and the promotion of ethical and professional conduct.

Canada
The Canadian health informatics association, known as COACH, has a membership ranging from health care executives, physicians, nurses and allied health professionals, researchers, and educators to Chief Information Officers, information managers, technical experts, consultants, and information technology vendors. COACH aims to promote understanding of health informatics within the Canadian health system.

New Zealand
Health Informatics New Zealand (HINZ) seeks to promote improvements in business processes and patient care through the application of appropriate information technologies. Membership is available to anyone with an interest in the New Zealand health informatics industry.

United Kingdom
The United Kingdom Council for Health Informatics Professions (UKCHIP) was formed in 2002 to promote professionalism in Health Informatics (HI). It operates a voluntary register of HI professionals who agree to work to clearly defined standards. Over 320 health informaticians

are now registered with UKCHIP and over 1400 more have started the registration process. The National Health Service recognises that 'Health Informatics encompasses a number of areas of knowledge and specialist activity where holding qualifications within a recognised professional framework is seen to be both appropriate and desirable' (National Health Service Information Authority 2001, p. 1).

USA

The American Medical Informatics Association (AMIA) represents individuals, institutions, and corporations involved in developing and using information technologies to improve health care.

BOX 2.5

ROLES FOR THE HEALTH INFORMATICS PROFESSIONAL

- Chief Information Officer, Chief Knowledge Officer
- Chief Medical Information Officer
- Clinical informatics professionals (nursing, medical, pharmacy etc.)
- Department/Middle Information Manager/Project Manager
- Information systems implementation (clinical and non-clinical)
- Information Management Specialist (non-management position)
- Information Security Manager/Officer
- Knowledge Manager
- Medical Records Manager
- Medical Records Administrator
- Medical Records/Librarian
- Health Information Technician

BOX 2.6

OPPORTUNITIES FOR HEALTH INFORMATICS PROFESSIONALS

- Hospitals and other health care providers
- Pharmaceutical companies
- Medical software companies
- Consulting companies
- Public health organisations
- Government and non-government agencies
- Insurance companies
- Academia

That these roles occur at all levels within organisations, and across many areas of endeavour indicates the increasingly central role of information management in health. In fact, health informatics skills are becoming essential for all health occupations. In 2001, the National Health Service in Great Britain published Health Informatics Competency Profiles for all professional staff. The URL for this list can be found in the WWW links at the end of the chapter. The specialist profession is evolving in conjunction with this broader trend.

The development of a profession involves both academics and professionals. The knowledge, skills, and accreditation process encapsulating a profession are generally linked to an academic discipline. The discipline shapes the profession, building knowledge through research, and disseminating that knowledge through the education of professionals. In turn, the profession shapes the discipline, as professional practice is frequently the source of research problems, issues, and the content of academic programs.

This is something of a problem for health informatics. As the boundaries of the discipline are somewhat fluid, so too are the boundaries of the profession. As Boxes 2.5 and 2.6 show, health informatics professionals are found in widely diverse clinical, technical, and administrative environments, undertaking management, service delivery, education, research, or support roles. This diversity indicates the breadth of opportunities available, which is exciting for the health informatics student. At the same time it creates some confusion: 'The vagueness has made it particularly difficult to argue that workers in medical informatics have special skills, since the boundaries of those skill sets are not identified' (Musen & van Bemmel 2002, p. 106). Some suggest that diversity makes it difficult to define health informatics as a distinct professional area and efforts are currently being directed towards identifying key skills and core content for health informatics education programs and accreditation processes.

On the other hand, diversity does produce a dynamic environment enabling many different perspectives to be presented and explored. The challenge is to find a way to incorporate these views into a coherent whole: 'The diversity of those working in health informatics brings a wide variety of viewpoints: we work together as health informaticians if we are to achieve the desired registered professional status' (Hayes 2000 in Taylor 2002, p. 3).

A BALANCING ACT

A further consideration is the variety of vested interests involved in the health care sector and the power they wield (Clarke 2001, p. 6).

Different groups and professions explore health informatics from their own perspective. While there may be general agreement regarding the overall goals and purpose of health informatics, different groups have different views about how this should be achieved and the priorities, problems, and solutions that are appropriate to the field. Views on the relative importance of privacy illustrate this. A report on *Research Challenges in E-Health Technologies* identified patient privacy as a primary issue for both research and the practice of health information management (Clarke 2001, p. 5).

Yet health executives responding to the Commonwealth Fund International Survey of Health Executives (2003) viewed privacy concerns as less of an issue than start-up costs, maintenance costs, and lack of standards (Table 2.3).

Table 2.3 Major barriers to greater use of computer technology

Per cent naming	Australia	Canada	New Zealand	UK	USA
High start-up costs	84	84	93	69	71
Projected maintenance costs	49	42	32	52	27
Lack of uniform standards	49	35	50	31	44
Privacy concerns	20	26	7	8	17

At the beginning of Part 1, it was noted that the health care environment is inherently political, with factions, pressure groups, and interest groups seeking to promote their own views and interests. This is also true of the field of health informatics. While the existence of these different perspectives may be positive, generating debate and increasing knowledge and understanding, it is important to realise that not all views will be equally represented. More powerful groups are able to exert more influence than marginal groups. This may see some issues ignored, some options not presented, and some solutions never considered. Research by Horsfield and Peterson (2000), which might usefully be applied to the discipline of health informatics, illustrates this. Through an analysis of key terms used to 'articulate policy, infrastructure priorities, deployment of technology, the design of health care services, investment and research', Horsfield and Peterson described and ranked 'key discourses that characterise contemporary E-Health diffusion practices in Australia'(2004, p. 1). Horsfield and Peterson suggest that Australia in 2000 was characterised by marginalised consumer and critical discourses, and a commerce-dominant discourse of e-health (and health informatics). Table 2.4 summarises the hierarchy.

The most powerful discourses are able to significantly shape the character and direction of health informatics, promoting some issues and activities and excluding others. Descriptions of policy, priority areas, and programs, and discussions of the advantages and disadvantages of various initiatives, point to the relative influence of different groups and their position within the power hierarchy. This may change over time as different values, assumptions, and priorities and different challenges and solutions come to the fore. This is seen in the initial domination of the technology discourse that declined somewhat as socio-technical-based clinical discourses became increasingly influential.

The success of many health informatics initiatives may depend upon how well different perspectives are acknowledged, negotiated, and integrated. 'It will be crucial for the health informatics field to account for the needs and concerns of all parties who participate in the process: patients, clinicians, payers and governments' (Hersh 2002, p. 1957).

Something of a balancing act is required, with compromises and trade-offs needing to be made. This is a challenge, particularly when key players do not have equal

Table 2.4 Discourses on e-health

Discourse	Focus
Technology discourse	Focuses on computing systems and technology. Contains an underlying assumption that technology will inevitably benefit all stakeholders in the health care system.
Administrator discourse	Views e-health in terms of efficiency, rationalisation, modernisation, and resource management.
Clinician discourse	Sees e-health in terms of patient care and patient outcomes. It represents the view of the health professional. The many different clinical and other groups of health professionals share the same broad orientation towards e-health.
Commercial discourse	Represents commerce and industry and uses the language of business. Commercialisation of e-health is an important issue for this group.
Academic discourse	The perspective of academics in the field of e-health.
Critical discourse	Views e-health in terms of power and control.
Consumer discourse	Talks about consumer participation, informed decision-making, and empowerment and represents the views and beliefs of those on the receiving end of health services.

Source: Horsfield and Peterson 2000, p. 6.

influence in shaping decisions within the health care system. One approach is to foster the development of a critical perspective within health informatics. A critical perspective need not be negative but would facilitate questions such as:

- How will the introduction of this system affect stakeholders?
- How will stakeholders view the introduction of this system?
- Who will be the main beneficiaries of this application/system?
- How will this application enable consumers to receive better health care and at what cost will this be achieved?

Health informatics professionals may have limited opportunity or inclination to dabble in the politics of influence. They will have the opportunity to explore their own perspective, which will shape their approach to their work. They may also have the opportunity to encourage dominant players to listen to the views of less dominant players. This is an integral element of a socio-technical approach to health informatics.

SUMMARY

Health informatics is concerned with the management of data, information, and knowledge in the health care environment. The discipline emerged from the broader discipline of informatics due to an interest in the management of health information and the particular demands of biomedical knowledge and the health care environment.

Since it emerged in the 1970s, health informatics has evolved from an initial focus on the use of computers and information technology in the management of medical information to a more broad ranging discipline with a multi-disciplinary base and application to a range of health and medical areas. This has included the broadening of the technology focus to a socio-technical focus incorporating cultural and organisational issues. Nevertheless, there is some criticism that technology issues continue to dominate, while other issues are given inadequate attention.

Within the academic arena, health informatics has not as yet developed an underlying theory but draws on theories from its multi-disciplinary base. Although utilising scientific method for research, health informatics has not itself established a strong methodological approach. This creates challenges in both defining the boundaries of the academic discipline and establishing a discrete profession with specialised knowledge and skills.

While the very breadth and inclusiveness of health informatics facilitates diversity and flexibility in both the identification of issues and solutions, it creates problems as the differing perspectives seek to shape the field according to their own priorities, issues, and solutions. The views of key players may not always be in agreement. One group may perceive advantage in an initiative, while others perceive disadvantage. This is significant for the health informatics professional, since the success of information management solutions is likely to be significantly influenced by the response of key players. It becomes a challenge since some groups are more able than others to have their views accepted. As part of a socio-technical stance, the health informatics professional will endeavour to identify the perspectives of key players, and where possible, seek solutions that attempt to balance these.

WWW LINKS

Professional associations and issues

International Medical Informatics Association (IMIA) <http://www.imia.org/>
Health Informatics Society of Australia (HISA) <http://www.hisa.org.au>
COACH: Canada's Health Informatics Association <http://www.coachorg.com>
Health Informatics New Zealand (HINZ) <http://www.hinz.org.nz/allabout/about.htm>
UK Council for Health Informatics Professions (UKCHIP) <http://www.ukchip.org/>
American Medical Informatics Association (AMIA) <http://www.amia.org>
Health Informatics Competency Profiles for the NHS, February 2001 <http://www.rcseng.ac.uk/dental/fds/training_pathway/pdf/hi_ecdl.pdf>
IMIA Code of Ethics <http://www.imia.org/code_of_ethics.html>

CRITICAL THINKING

The community nurses and allied health professionals working out of the Global Village Community Health Centre are seeking to improve information sharing as they work together to support older residents with chronic health problems. Currently, the community nurses and each allied health area maintain their own records, and information is shared at case conferences. Much of this information could be more efficiently communicated using a database management system, which would allow health professionals to merge and share their data and information. The database will be located on the Centre server, and each professional will access the data from their own workstation.

1   What are the characteristics of this scenario that point to a need for a health informatics professional to develop solutions?

2   From a technology perspective, what might be the key questions? From a problem focus, what might be the key questions?

3   Who might be the key stakeholders in this environment and what might their priorities be? What might be their concerns?

4   The system is to be evaluated in terms of efficiency and usability. What research approaches might be appropriate and what questions might be asked?

CHAPTER 3

BUILDING THE KNOWLEDGE BASE

OVERVIEW

Health informatics has established itself as an applied discipline focusing on the practical problems of information management in the health care environment. To do this it draws on the concepts and theories of other disciplines, rather than develop its own. These include the disciplines of education, sociology, social psychology, computing, and information technology. Drawing on other disciplines has definite advantages for facilitating diversity and flexibility in identifying, exploring, and solving issues. It also helps to ensure the relevance of health informatics to the many different environments and professions in health care. This chapter is a general overview of the concepts and theories utilised by health informatics. It is intended to complement, rather than replace, the detailed analyses and discussions found in the disciplines from which these concepts and theories are drawn.

OBJECTIVES

At the completion of this chapter, you should be able to:
- define key concepts used in health informatics
- outline theories used in health informatics
- use examples to demonstrate how these concepts and theories contribute to the practice of health informatics.

CONCEPTS AND THEORIES

Model

Systems theory

Information

Learning theory

Information technology

Adult learning theory

Security

Diffusion of innovation theory

Usability

Change management theory

Organisation

Positivist social science

Culture and subculture

Interpretive social science

Status, roles, and power

Critical social science

INTRODUCTION

> The discipline utilises the methods and technologies of the information sciences for the purposes of problem solving and decision-making thus assuring quality health care in all basic and applied areas of biomedical sciences for the community it serves (HISA 2004).

This chapter discusses the concepts and theories used to develop the knowledge base and inform the practice of health informatics. It begins by reviewing the role of concepts and theories in the development of a social science discipline. It then focuses on a number of concepts drawn from disciplines contributing to health informatics. These concepts are used to explore phenomena in the social environment. A number of these are also an integral element of the theories used in health informatics. The final section of the chapter discusses several of these theories. The concepts and theories are introduced rather than explored in great detail; more in-depth information and debate should be sought in specialised texts and resources.

THE BUILDING BLOCKS

Building scientific knowledge is a continuous process of observation, questioning, proposing tentative explanations, and testing those explanations. The building blocks of this process are concepts, hypotheses, and theories. In practice these terms often overlap, making it somewhat artificial to separate them. At the same time, separating them does help to distinguish between them, and explain their role in the knowledge-building process.

Revisiting the knowledge-building process

The process of building knowledge using scientific method begins with the observation of some natural or social phenomena. If the phenomena are unusual or if the observer has an enquiring mind, he or she might begin to ask what, how, and why questions. If the observer is imaginative, as well as curious, he or she might then begin to develop tentative explanations. If the observer has been trained in scientific methods, these explanations will be framed in such a way that they are testable. The explanation will be in the form of a hypothesis. Being trained in the scientific method, the observer will seek to make the hypothesis clear and concise.

If the observer is fortunate enough to have the resources, the next step in building knowledge will be to conduct research to establish whether or not the hypothesis can be supported. This, of course, will involve the collection of data or evidence according to clearly defined rules, procedures, and techniques. If the evidence provides strong support for the hypothesis, it may become part of the body of knowledge of the discipline. It will either add to our understanding of existing theories, or if the knowledge is significant, become a new theory in its own right. A hypothesis that is not supported may still contribute to the knowledge base of the discipline. Rather than create new knowledge, an unsupported hypothesis supports existing knowledge. Box 3.1 is an example of the knowledge-building process.

BOX 3.1

BUILDING KNOWLEDGE

In the early 1980s, doctors noticed that an unusually high number of young gay men in New York and California were developing a rare type of pneumonia and a rare form of cancer known as Kaposi's sarcoma. As these conditions did not usually occur in young gay men, doctors became concerned and began to investigate. They began to ask what, why, and how questions. For example, what symptoms were these men displaying? Why were they occurring in this group of men? How could they set about explaining this unusual phenomenon? Scientists quickly began to find answers to these questions, establishing the existence of HIV and AIDS. Key links appeared to be the role of bath houses and the transmission of HIV. This was linked to data about the experiences of men who developed AIDS, to existing knowledge about the transmission of water-borne disease, and to the sexual practices of gay men who frequented these bath houses. One hypothesis that was proposed was that the disease was spread through the water in the bath houses, while another hypothesised that sexual practices were linked to transmission. Both hypotheses suggested a causal relationship. The hypothesis that HIV could be transmitted through water was shown to be false. While sexual practices among gay men appeared to be associated with the transmission of HIV, it was eventually shown to be a blood-borne virus that could infect a range of people in a number of different ways. These findings have now become part of the biomedical knowledge base.

CONCEPTS

A **concept**, expressed as a symbol or a word, is a shorthand way of representing an idea. Email, for example, is shorthand for 'a messaging system available on computer networks, providing users with personal mail-boxes from which electronic messages can be sent and received' (Coiera 2003, p. 400). Concepts represent both concrete ideas such as data, and abstract ideas such as knowledge.

We use concepts in everyday life. Clusters of concepts also form specialised languages or **jargon**. Most fields of endeavour have a specialised language that evolves as the field itself grows. We see this in the many new concepts that have emerged as information and communications technologies have developed. Concepts within a discipline may be drawn from prior research, existing theories, or may be coined during new research. Health informatics, as an applied discipline, has tended to draw on other fields and disciplines for its concepts. The obvious exception is the concept 'informatics', which, as we have seen, was coined to describe a new science. The following concepts will be useful for exploring and applying health informatics within a socio-technical perspective.

Models

Model is a concept widely utilised in health informatics. Talman and Hasman (2003, p. 211) describe health informatics as a 'modelling discipline', while Coiera (2003, p. 3) refers to the model as the pivotal concept of health informatics.

A model can be a small physical copy or representation of an object, such as a model boat or car, or it can be a pictorial or diagrammatic representation as shown in Figure 3.1, which is a model representing the physical layout of a small suburban general practice.

Figure 3.1 Model of general practice surgery

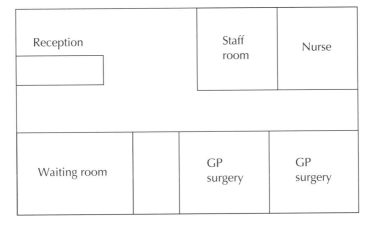

Models can also represent abstract processes such as workflow in an emergency department, a financial model for an electronic health record or, as in Figure 3.2, the movement of a patient through the GP surgery.

Figure 3.2 Patient-movement model

Step 1   Check with reception
Step 2   Wait
Step 3   Complete paperwork
Step 4   Proceed to waiting room
Step 5   Wait
Step 6   Proceed to GP consulting room
Step 7   Wait
Step 8   Return to reception
Step 9   Wait
Step 10 Pay
Step 11 Leave building

Models represent objects and processes visually as a plan, diagram, or flow chart, or as a list of steps as shown in Figure 3.2. Visual representation helps to structure and organise our thinking about abstract, often complex, entities. It also enables us to analyse and manipulate the entity or process. This then facilitates manipulation and modification of the entity or process in the real world.

Models of existing objects or processes are not generally exact replicas. They are somewhat simplified with some detail omitted. The model of the general practice surgery does not include all of the furniture and fittings, while the model of patient movements does not include the actions of health professionals.

The decision about what to include or exclude in a model depends upon the purpose of the model and the assumptions or view of the creator. This means that, depending on the purpose of the model, the same object or process may produce quite different models. A cost–benefit model of an electronic health record will differ markedly from a clinical model. Neither model can be considered as more accurate than the other. They simply represent different views.

Models may also be templates for planned objects or processes. These too are based on assumptions and perspectives, in this case about the proposed uses of the object or process. The physicians in a general practice may be planning to install a small information system that requires a model of the data flow through the practice. The designer of the system might assume that the reception staff will enter all data and information, or that the physicians will enter all data and information, or that the reception staff will enter administrative data and the physicians will enter all clinical data. (What about the nurse?) These different assumptions will produce quite different data flow models.

The accuracy of assumptions will impact on the usefulness of the system that is created from a model.

Data, information, knowledge

In Chapter 2, it was noted that the concept *information* encapsulates the field of health informatics. Information is a complex concept often represented as the interrelated concepts of data, information, and knowledge. Box 3.2 defines these concepts and identifies the basic relationships between them.

Health informatics seeks to uncover the relationships between health data, information, and knowledge, and apply them to the analysis and resolution of information management problems. The concepts and their relationship are therefore fundamental to health informatics.

The concepts can be applied at the individual level, as in Box 3.2, where the health professional interprets the temperature data and information for individual patients. They can also be applied at the domain or discipline level as shown in Box 3.3.

Shaping knowledge

> Where does medical knowledge come from and where ought it to come from? (Georgiou 2002, p. 127).

Chapters 1 and 2 have noted that rational science endeavours to produce objective knowledge. Yet the production of scientific knowledge can be mediated by the specific

BOX 3.2

RELATIONSHIP BETWEEN DATA, INFORMATION, AND KNOWLEDGE

- Data generally refers to raw facts as in descriptions, observations, images, or sounds. A simple example is the numbers 39.5, 37.5, and 38.5. These numbers have no context or meaning. These are data.
- Data that is interpreted, organised, or structured in a meaningful way becomes information. For example, if the numbers 39.5, 37.5, and 38.5 were to be arranged and presented as the temperature pattern, in degrees Centigrade, over the past twelve hours for a given hospital patient, we have information. Adding meaning to data creates information.
- Bringing understanding to information produces knowledge. In our example, the health care professional uses rules, relationships, and past experiences in drawing conclusions about the patient's temperature and deciding on a course of action.

BOX 3.3

DOMAIN LEVEL DATA, INFORMATION, AND KNOWLEDGE

Domain level data might be:
- diet records of a group of heart patients
- exercise records of the group
- weight records of the group
- family history of heart disease for the group.
  This data could be organised as information to show:
- relationships between diet, exercise, and heart disease
- possible family links in heart disease.
  Analysis of this information might result in the knowledge that excessive weight, a fatty diet, and lack of exercise are factors contributing to a high risk of heart disease. This knowledge might be used to:
- educate people about healthy lifestyles and health risks
- improve treatment options.
  This knowledge might then become part of the biomedical knowledge base.

social, economic, and political environment in which it occurs. Funding bodies can select some issues for research and ignore others, while the results of research can be interpreted differentially. This is seen in past and current debates around the effects of tobacco, asbestos, and global warming. Georgiou (2002, p. 129) argues that the informatics model of data, information, and knowledge has the potential to allow this influence to occur. He views this model as simplistic and argues that the method by which data becomes knowledge is 'a much more involved process, a product of intense scientific debate, successes and failures'. Adoption of the informatics model can therefore lead to a distortion of scientific research (see Box 3.4).

If health informatics is not to become simply a tool of 'politicians, bureaucrats and their statistical technicians' (Charlton & Miles 1998, in Georgiou 2002, p. 129), some understanding of the complexity of knowledge and knowledge management will be useful.

BOX 3.4

DISTORTING RESEARCH?

Governments and health insurers are attracted to the notion of allocating 'cost-effective' health resources on the basis of 'evidence'. There are many difficulties involved in resource allocation, however, and often the large quantities of trial data required to meet the standards of evidence simply do not exist. The effect of this may be a systematic bias towards treatments in areas where there are existing funds available to show effectiveness (for example, new pharmaceutical agents) at the expense of other areas where rigorous evidence does not currently exist or is not easily attainable (Kerridge et al. 1998, cited in Georgiou 2002, p. 127).

Knowledge management

While knowledge management may be viewed as part of the data–information–knowledge continuum, knowledge itself, as discussed above, is more than a complex type of information that can be neatly stored in a database. Knowledge requires intuition, judgment, perhaps wisdom, to make sense of and use data and information. Knowledge can be defined along several dimensions, including:

- *Explicit and tacit knowledge*: **Explicit knowledge** is formal and structured, can be expressed verbally and can be easily transmitted to others. **Tacit or implicit knowledge** is unstructured, or loose. It derives from personal experience and involves subjective insight, intelligence, and intuition. It is more difficult to communicate since it resides in people's minds and they may not have articulated it to themselves. Much medical knowledge is tacit. This is why it is described as fuzzy.
- *Individual knowledge and organisational knowledge*: **Individual knowledge** is manifested through individual skills or expertise. A nurse, for example, possesses tacit and explicit knowledge about nursing care, which is manifested through

patient care activities and interaction with other professionals. **Organisational knowledge** is collective knowledge. An individual possesses only a subset of organisational knowledge. In a hospital, staff physicians may provide medical expertise for diagnosis and treatment, but they may have little or no familiarity with patient billing, resource allocation, or other aspects of health care administration.

* *Social knowledge and structured knowledge*: Organisational knowledge may be either social knowledge or structured knowledge. Social knowledge is knowledge shared by groups within the organisation. It is largely tacit, and develops only as a result of working together. An example of tacit social knowledge is the understanding that various health-professional groups have of the way they relate to each other and their patients. Structured knowledge is generally explicit knowledge, embedded in an organisation's systems, processes, tools, and routines. It is often expressed in the form of policies, rules, and procedures.

Knowledge management seeks to make implicit knowledge explicit. This is a challenge, since knowledge, particularly tacit knowledge, is vague, dynamic, and constantly evolving and no database will adequately capture or maintain knowledge. Nor will an expert system ever replace an expert.

In the health sector, decision support and expert systems focus on knowledge management for management and clinical decision-making. The first challenge for such systems is to define and represent knowledge in an accessible form. This is discussed in Chapter 9.

Information technology

Very few texts define 'information technology'. Perhaps it is assumed to be self-explanatory. Yet the concept creates misconceptions about the focus of health informatics, while at the same time encapsulating a fundamental tool of the field.

The term 'information technology' refers to computer hardware, software, and communications technology used for the input, storage, processing, and communication of information. Communication includes voice, data, network, and satellite technology. This definition does not include processes or people, which distinguishes information technology from information systems. Information systems incorporate people, processes, and information technology. This distinction enables us to clearly identify the parameters of information technology and emphasise that it is an enabling tool, not the focus, of health informatics.

Security

Security is a key concern and therefore a key concept for health informatics. With the increasing integration of information systems and widespread adoption of electronic technologies, security is becoming an increasingly significant issue. The aim of security is to maintain the privacy, confidentiality, integrity, and availability of data.

Guidance for making security decisions can come from two places. One is the relevant national standards, such as Australian standard HB 174-2003, AS 13335 (set) 2003, and the other is the organisation's own security policies or business rules.

However, health organisations need to consider carefully the issue of privacy, as there is an inherent conflict between keeping data confidential and keeping it available. On the one hand, there is a need for access to data to make clinical decisions, while on the other hand, people may want to restrict access to data that they feel is essentially private and that may reflect badly upon them in some contexts.

Privacy and confidentiality

One of the biggest security issues is the need to protect the privacy of personal data. Privacy legislation in many countries now mandates how personally identified data (PID) must be managed. Box 3.5 lists some relevant legislation. For more detailed information, see the WWW links at the end of the chapter.

BOX 3.5 PRIVACY LEGISLATION

Australia
The *Privacy Act* 1998 (Cth) embodies principles for privacy based on the OECD ten principles for the use of personally identified data (PID) by governments. The Act was amended in 2000 to create principles that apply to the private sector and also health-related organisations. As the privacy of health-related data is of special concern there is whole section of the government privacy website devoted to how these principles apply.

Canada
The laws relating to privacy and health data are more complicated in Canada. This is because there is the overarching Canadian law, the *Personal Information and Electronic Documents Act* 2000, as well as individual province legislation. For example, Ontario has just passed a *Personal Health Information Protection Act* 2004 and British Columbia an amendment to its *Freedom of Information and Protection of Privacy Act* to deal with issues relating to the US *Patriot Act* and the fact that the management of their medical records is outsourced to US-owned companies.

New Zealand
The New Zealand Privacy Act 1993 is again based on the OECD 1980 Privacy Principles. It has been modified by the 1994 Health Information Privacy Code. This has been designed to help the health sector to meet the objectives of the Privacy Act by, for example, using language tailored to refer to the health sector. The Code takes precedence over the principles laid down in the Act and in general provides more stringent conditions. The New Zealand Privacy website contains a helpful overview of the Code as fact sheet number 10 (see WWW links).

United Kingdom

Again the United Kingdom legislation is derived from the OECD principles and is embodied in the *Data Protection Act* 1998. Guidance on the application of this act for the use and disclosure of data was issued in a comprehensive document in 2002.

USA

In the USA the *Health Insurance Portability and Accountability Act* (HIPAA) of 1996 requires that access to health information be tightly controlled. However, the Standards for Privacy of Individually Identifiable Health Information, issued by the US Department of Health and Human Services, establishes a set of national standards for the protection of certain health data. These aim to 'assure that individuals' health information is properly protected while allowing the flow of health information needed to provide and promote high quality health care and to protect the public's health and well being'.

Personally identifiable data or **personally identified information (PII)** is data containing details that enables it to be easily traced back to a particular individual. Health information systems deal with a great deal of this type of data. Maintaining confidentiality to the level desired is a problem for all information systems that manage PID. It is a particularly difficult problem for systems that operate in a health care environment due to the many competing demands for data across a wide spectrum of changing locations and personnel. There are different views about who should have access to each kind of personally identified health data.

Privacy and confidentiality

Privacy refers to the right of an individual to limit access to personal information. Confidentiality refers to 'the expectation that the information collected will be used for the purpose for which it was gathered' (Bialorucki & Blane 1992, in Johns 2002, p. 320). 'Purpose of use' is fundamental for all data held in information systems and was enunciated as the first requirement of the OECD principles. Health and medical data and information is particularly sensitive since it has the potential to be misused if made available, or accessed, for purposes other than that for which it was collected. Box 3.6 has examples of breaches of privacy and confidentiality of health and medical information.

Integrity

Integrity deals with consistency and accuracy of data and information. It focuses on preventing data from being incorrectly created or altered. Maintaining the integrity of health information begins with developing processes and templates that ensure the

BREACHES OF PRIVACY AND CONFIDENTIALITY

The University of Washington Medical Center information system was infiltrated and confidential information on thousands of patients was downloaded. The medical records contained information that could be used for identity theft. In another incident in the USA, 5000 administrative patient files were hacked from one of the country's top hospitals. Not all attacks necessarily come from the outside. Kropp and Gallaher (2001) reported that a significant number of organisations have experienced internal security lapses.

accurate and complete collection of data. Most electronic systems these days carefully check the integrity of each piece of data as it is entered. Electronic systems also use techniques to prevent data from being altered or deleted by unauthorised people. These include alerts, access privileges, and backup systems.

Availability

Availability refers to information being available when and where it is needed. There are three aspects to availability. The first is concerned with ensuring that authenticated users are able to access the relevant data and information. Passwords and PIN numbers are common methods for authentication. In an environment where many people may share computers and the user population is fluid, it can be very difficult to implement such a system. If access to data is to be restricted to enforce confidentiality requirements, then each user needs to be identified as they use the computer. In addition it is often required that users be sufficiently identified in order to have access to their own digital signing credentials. So, for example, a doctor who can authorise medications needs to be identified as someone different from the nurse who just accessed the care plan that indicates the need for such medication.

The second aspect of availability is preventing, detecting, and responding to attacks on computing infrastructure before such attacks can cause harm. Detection is a relatively new aspect of computer security that recognises that the best efforts at preventing attacks do not always work. Intrusion detection systems (IDS) monitor the activity on hosts and networks and try to work out when this activity matches or indicates that the system is being attacked.

The third role is the traditional one of setting systems in place so that if an attack is successful, essential functionality can be resumed as soon as possible with a full return to service achieved via a planned series of responses. The familiar techniques of backup and recovery are part of an integrated disaster recovery plan (often known by a more positive title of 'business continuity').

Risk assessment

One approach to managing security issues is to view them in the context of a risk-management strategy. There are three broad classes of risk that apply to all information management systems. These relate to:

- countering threats to operating ability and reputation
- complying with legal requirements
- fulfilling duty of care obligations.

The aim of risk assessment is to quantify the particular threats that a health care information system is exposed to and the potential impact of those threats. The Australian and New Zealand standard 4360:2004 provides a good description of the processes, decision aids, and tools involved in risk management. Tables 3.1 and 3.2 show how the matrix can be used to assess the potential impact of a threat and the potential for that threat to eventuate and the consequent priority for the organisation in managing the threat.

Table 3.1 Impact assessment

	Extreme	Major	Moderate	Minor	Insignificant
Ability to provide service					

Table 3.2 Threat potential and priority level

	Extreme	Major	Moderate	Minor	Insignificant
Almost certain	Top priority	Top priority	Top priority	Second priority	Second priority

Usability

Usability falls within the discipline of human–computer interaction and is concerned with how easy an application is to learn and to operate. The concept refers to every aspect of an information system with which a person interacts. Usability therefore includes hardware, software, menus, icons, messages, documentation, training, and online help. Usability can be considered in terms of three dimensions:

- **Product attributes:** factors such as screen layout, menus, and consistency.
- **User orientation:** explores user attributes, perceptions, and the environments within which users will be running a particular application.
- **User performance:** seeks to establish how well the product meets the task requirements.

Usability is an aspect of health information systems that was neglected for many years. It has now been acknowledged that it is an essential component in the success or failure of systems. Unfortunately, if Darbyshire's observation that 'clinicians' experiences were characterized by digital disappointment rather than electronic efficiencies' (2004, p. 17) is anything to go by, there is quite a lot of work still to be done. Usability is revisited in later chapters.

Sociological concepts

A socio-technical perspective seeks to understand the cultural and organisational aspects of information management. Sociology studies social structures and social interaction between individuals. Therefore, a number of sociological concepts are useful for understanding cultural and organisational aspects of the health environment. Concepts included here are:

- organisation
- culture and **subculture**
- structure
- status, roles, and power.

Organisation

Many health services are delivered within large and small organisations. An organisation is a group of people in a stable hierarchy of clearly defined roles and responsibilities, working together to achieve a common goal. Organisations develop their own culture and structure, and are differentiated from the wider society by defined boundaries.

Culture and subculture

The culture of an organisation includes its shared values and attitudes, norms, and climate.

- Values and attitudes express what is important within the organisation. For example, your health organisation might value professional growth and the use of initiative and teamwork, or it might value tradition, conforming to established professional relationships, and following policies and protocols.
- Norms are rules or guidelines for acceptable behaviour within the organisation. Norms can be both formal, such as protocols for dispensing drugs, and informal, such as ways of addressing particular groups of staff.
- The **organisational climate** is shaped by the values and attitudes of the organisation. It is the 'atmosphere' of the workplace. An organisation may have a climate that encourages tradition and routine, or it may have a climate that supports experimentation and trying new ways of working. The climate is how you 'feel' about your work environment.

Most organisations, particularly larger ones, have subcultures. These are variations from the main culture. They develop where people perform similar functions, or share the same professional occupation. In a large hospital there may be a nursing subculture, a subculture shared by allied health professionals, or a subculture shared by the information technology department. Professional subcultures have their own area of knowledge and expertise, their own particular interests and their own agendas. The more diverse the subcultures in an organisation, the wider the range of self-interests will be, and the greater the possibility that the interests of one group may be adversely affected by those of other subcultures.

The health care environment has traditionally been characterised by strong professional subcultures, many of which are very protective of their knowledge and sphere of influence. Biomedical professional subcultures have been evolving since the emergence of scientific medicine and the modern hospital.

In recent years, there have been a number of pressures on these silo subcultures. These include patient empowerment (with its accompanying scepticism of biomedical authority), clinical governance and the increasing inroads being made by information management systems. Information management systems have the potential to cut across professional boundaries, thus impacting on established roles and relationships. The resistance of many health professionals, particularly clinicians, to information systems can be partly explained by this challenge. If the new system requires an adjustment of roles and practices, then there may be user resistance.

A socio-technical perspective will be cognisant of the professional subcultures, their potential influence on the introduction of information systems, and the impact that these systems may in turn have on professional subcultures.

Structure

Organisations develop a structure to enable them to carry out activities and functions. The structure defines roles and responsibilities, their span of authority, and communication channels. Once established, the structure changes very slowly. It was noted in Chapter 1 that health organisations have generally adopted a traditional bureaucratic structure. Characteristics of this structure include:

- *Pyramid shape*: Fewer individuals are at the higher levels than at the lower levels. Higher levels generally have higher status.
- *Chain of command*: Power and authority are vested in the higher levels and delegated to lower levels, and this is clearly identifiable.
- *Communication channels*: These are based on the hierarchy of authority, and are vertical rather than horizontal.
- *Emphasis on routine and conformity*: Written policies, protocols, and processes define how members conduct their daily activities and interactions.

In the health environment, two trends in organisation structures have been identified. The first, discussed in Chapter 1, is the trend towards the increasing complexity of bureaucratic structures with multiple lines of power and authority, and the increased potential for tension and conflict as professional subcultures seek to further their own agenda. The second trend is towards flatter, more democratic structures that facilitate increased participation in management, teamwork, horizontal rather than vertical communication, and less rigid routines and processes. In today's large, complex health systems, variations of both types of structures will often exist within the one organisation. Box 3.7 describes a typical health care organisation.

BOX 3.7 TYPICAL CONTEMPORARY HEALTH CARE ORGANISATION

This regional health care organisation is large and complex and characterised by the typical hierarchical structure, including autocratic, centralised decision-making on issues affecting the organisation as a whole. It consists of four sections: Strategic and Corporate Services, Health Promotion, Community Health, and Hospitals Services. The four sections work within the broad parameters of Health Department policy but exercise a degree of autonomy over structure and management processes in their area. Hospitals Services closely reflect the structure of the organisation as a whole, but other divisions have flatter, more democratic management structures and team-based operations.

Status, roles, and power

Status refers to a position in a social structure, in this case, the organisation. Characteristics used to confer status can include age, gender, ethnicity, and occupation. In a health care organisation, status is generally based on education and occupation or profession. In large complex organisations there may be multiple status hierarchies. Power can vary in accordance to status. There is also a set of expectations, or a role, defining how the person occupying that status should act. Roles include obligations and privileges. Status and roles are reciprocal. Finally, roles are not rigid, but are generally viewed as guidelines. Over time they change. Box 3.8 illustrates these properties.

Roles evolve slowly, and sudden changes may be resisted, particularly if the changes are imposed by others. The introduction of health information systems and technologies into a health organisation frequently results in changes to established roles and relationships. This is thought to be one reason for the limited acceptance of so many systems: 'Organisationally, new clinical information systems alter traditional practice and workflow...distribution of resources and power may be affected...physicians may resist if they perceive that medical diagnoses will be degraded, or if their work roles, status, or autonomy will be adversely affected' (Tanriverdi & Iacono 1999, p. 225).

BOX 3.8

ROLES, STATUS, POWER

Status is associated with power. The Queen of England has a great deal more power than the unemployed teenager. The brain surgeon has more power than the student nurse. Generally, the higher the status in the hierarchy, the more power there is attached to that status.

Status includes obligations and privileges. The Queen of England is expected to attend official functions, wear her tiara, and not get roaring drunk. Her privileges include the use of a range of luxurious palaces, yachts and jets, respect from lesser persons, and precedence. The heart surgeon is expected to show up at the operating theatre and perform intricate and expensive operations. Privileges might include relative autonomy, respect, and high monetary rewards. The student nurse is expected to care for patients and study the relevant domain knowledge. The privilege will be acquiring a qualification.

Status and role are reciprocal. For the status of Queen, there will be a reciprocal status of subject. For the status of physician, there will be a reciprocal status of patient. The student nurse and the lecturer are reciprocal roles.

Roles evolve over time. At one time, it was acceptable for the monarch to get roaring drunk and lop people's heads off. It was not acceptable for student nurses to go out at night, drink alcohol, or get married.

THEORIES

> Investigators in any area of science require theories that can frame the interpretation of observations and that can provide the basis for making advances in understanding (Musen & van Bemmel. 2003, p. 217).

A theory is used to explain what the physical or social world is like, how that world changes and/or why it changes. As an applied discipline, health informatics has focused on solving the practical problems in the health care environment, drawing on the theories of other disciplines, rather than developing its own.

Systems theory

> Rather than reducing an entity (e.g. the human body) to the properties of its parts or elements (e.g. organs or cells), systems theory focuses on the arrangement of and relations between the parts which connect them into a whole (Heylighen & Joslyn 1992, p. 1).

Systems theory has long been used by biomedical science as a means of explaining and understanding the entities and processes of health care. The physiology of the human body is discussed in terms of skeletal system, muscular system, nervous system, and so on. Health informatics has also adopted a systems approach to assist in understanding and managing the flow of health information.

General systems theory evolved in the mid-twentieth century within the biological and physical sciences. Until this time, the approach to understanding complex organisms such as the human body was to examine individual component parts. Each system within the human body would be isolated and the components examined. This approach is reflected in the structuring of biomedical knowledge, which, as has been discussed, was typically organised into specialties and subspecialties.

General systems theory focuses on the system as a whole. Advocates argue that complex organisms are better understood by studying not only individual components, but also the ways the individual parts interact and affect each other. Today systems theory is utilised by many disciplines, including medicine, engineering, computing, information systems, and sociology.

Before discussing the characteristics of systems, it is perhaps worth noting that health organisations are also now routinely referred to as health systems rather than services. The meaning of the term in reference to health systems, however, does not necessarily imply the integrated and connected characteristics of systems discussed here.

A system

Systems theory views complex organisms such as the human body as 'a whole[:]...their components or parts, their attributes or characteristics, can only be understood as a function of the total system' (Ruegger & Johns 1992, p. 10). Systems may be living, non-living, or a combination of both. In the health care environment, the majority of systems consist of living (people) and non-living (information, technology) components. They are socio-technical systems.

Systems can include subsystems, which are themselves systems. A health system may include hospitals, nursing homes, and community centres, which are all subsystems of the health system, yet they are systems in their own right. Similarly, a health information system may include a pharmacy information subsystem, a nursing information subsystem, and a financial information subsystem.

Figure 3.3 GP system and subsystem

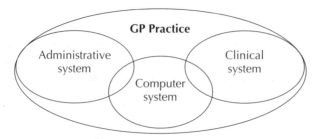

Figure 3.3 shows the GP practice discussed earlier as a system composed of sub-systems. For simplicity the figure includes only three subsystems, although it is possible to use more (or less) depending on the perspective from which the system is viewed.

Boundaries and environments

Systems are located within a particular environment. A system is separated from its environment by a boundary, which may be permeable or impermeable. An impermeable boundary results in a closed system allowing no interaction with the surrounding environment. There are very few closed systems. Most systems are open, with semi-permeable boundaries, allowing interaction with the environment. The environment influences the way an open system operates, and the interaction between the system and the environment is not always predictable. As a consequence of interaction with the environment, systems can acquire new characteristics and properties. Figure 3.4 illustrates the environment within which the GP system exists.

Understanding system boundaries assists in the development of information systems by defining the scope of the system. The boundary defines which information is in and which information is out of the system.

Figure 3.4 A system and its environment

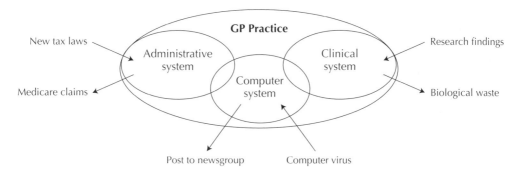

2 + 2 = 5

The individual parts of a system cannot do what the system as a whole can do. While each individual part may perform particular activities even in isolation, it is the combination of these parts into a unified whole that makes a system. Once combined, the parts of the system interrelate in a structured way that differs from the activities of the individual components. Five basketball players on a court can each dribble the ball and shoot baskets. Once they take up positions, support each other, and begin to pass the ball around, they become a team (system) and in doing so they become more than five individuals. Similarly, individual health professionals do not become a team (system) until they begin to interact, communicate, and exchange information. Without established relationships there is no system, just a group of individuals. Health information systems are often classified according to their purpose, so that we have a radiology system, an order entry system, a pharmacy system, or a human resource management system.

Following from this is the assumption that systems are goal-directed. Systems exist for a purpose. Individual system components combine to cooperate in achieving goals.

Inputs, processes, outputs

The key features of a system are inputs, processes, and outputs. The system accepts inputs, which it processes in some way before returning them to the environment. Patients enter a hospital (inputs), are treated (processes), and leave the hospital (outputs).

Where a number of systems are arranged as a series, the output of one becomes the input for another. This is demonstrated in Figure 3.5, where a car crash victim enters hospital and is treated (processed) through various hospital systems.

Figure 3.5 A series of systems

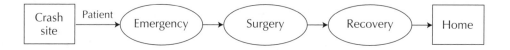

Systems and change

Systems persist over a period of time and, once established, tend to resist change. At the same time open systems exist in, and interact with, dynamic environments. They need to respond to changes in the external environment if they are to continue to achieve their goals. If they cannot adapt, they become non-functional. This means that systems are in a constant state of change or adjustment to changes in the environment. The general practice system may change in response to changes in reporting and reimbursement arrangements, the introduction of a pharmacy-practice information system, or even a change in the characteristics of patients using the practice.

Generally, changes are small and are a part of the evolution of the system. Sometimes changes are larger and may upset the balance of the system. Since the components of a system interact, a change in one part of the system will impact on all other parts of the system.

Systems theory and health informatics

In today's health care environment, information flows within and between health organisations in increasingly complex ways. A multitude of systems collect, manipulate, and communicate information to inform decisions ranging from routine administrative processes to obscure clinical diagnoses. Systems theory provides a framework for understanding and managing this information flow. Using systems theory, together with modelling techniques, we are able to trace the flow of information within an organisation, region, state, or even national health system, and identify how information within individual parts and/or subsystems interacts with and affects other parts of the system. Using the concept of boundaries, we can identify subsystems within an organisation, the information requirements specific to each system, and the interchange across systems. The concepts of inputs, processes, and outputs enable us to specify the required data, manipulations, and information to be produced for individual systems. Finally, systems theory allows us to explore the potential impact of change on a system and its environment.

Since health care organisations are complex socio-technical systems, health-informatics professionals need to draw on additional theories to complement the understanding achieved from applying systems theory to the health care environment.

Learning theories

The field of teaching and learning

Learning can be defined as an increase in knowledge, a change in attitude or values, the development of new skills, or the application of any of these in a new situation. Learning can be formal or informal and can involve both tacit and explicit knowledge. Clearly, this is a complex area. As with so many of the social sciences, there are a number of different theories and perspectives about how and why people learn. The online Theory into Practice Database lists more than fifty theories, together with a range of learning domains and concepts. While there may be some debate between supporters of various perspectives, it is generally accepted that each theory contributes to the overall understanding of learning and learning processes.

Learning theories

Learning theories seek to explain how learning occurs and what influences the process. Theories seeking to explain influences on the learning process often draw on the linked concepts of motivation and reinforcement. Motivation is the desire to learn, while reinforcement is the feedback the learner receives during or after learning. Positive reinforcement is considered to motivate the learner to continue, whereas negative reinforcement motivates the learner to discontinue. The foundations for many of these theories are **behaviourism** (external motivation) and **humanism** (internal motivation and self-actualisation).

Learning theories also seek to explain how the learning process occurs in the brain. These **cognitive learning** theories focus on cognitive processes in the brain. Table 3.3 summarises these approaches.

Contemporary learning theories

Contemporary theories and perspectives often adopt a relative view of learning, drawing on other theories to develop an understanding of individual learner characteristics and learning styles, domains, and environments.

Table 3.3 Perspectives on learning

Perspective	Theorists	View of learning
Behaviourism	Pavlov Skinner Thorndike Guthrie	These are psychological theories that explain learning in terms of conditioning and that regard learning in terms of what can be objectively observed and measured.
Cognitive theories	Dewey Vygotsky Piaget	The cognitive perspective assumes that learning occurs at a cognitive level, and may or may not involve observable behaviour. It suggests that learning occurs when incoming information can be related to existing knowledge in the brain, then stored where it can be retrieved when needed. Cognitive theories influenced the field of learning styles.
Humanism	Knowles Rogers Maslow	Humanists view learning as synonymous with personal growth and therefore assume that people naturally want to learn, that they are internally motivated, and that they are best able to decide for themselves what and how they should learn. The learner is viewed as an active participant who learns through a series of inter-personal relationships and will not learn if he or she does not want to.
Social learning	Gagne	Reinforcement and shaping of responses are important factors in social learning.

Andragogy, for example, which is probably the most widely known adult learning theory, includes concepts from behaviourism, humanism, and cognitive theory. The theory suggests that adults:

- need reasons for learning
- need to learn by experience
- approach learning as problem solving
- learn best when the topic is of immediate value.

There are a number of comprehensive resources on learning theory. A very good contemporary discussion with a health focus is that by Eraut in Coffield's *Differing Visions of a Learning Society* (2000).

Learning theories have a number of applications in health informatics. Application of learning theories will:

- enhance usability by informing the design of user interfaces and system processes
- facilitate the development of the education and training component of systems implementation

- enhance the quality of online education programs, which are increasingly a part of the health care environment.

ORGANISATIONS AND CHANGE

Health care organisations are systems, comprising people, data, processes, and technology. Information systems are subsystems of health care organisations. Changes to health information systems will affect all component parts of the system and the reactions of people to these changes cannot always be predicted or controlled. Theories of innovation and change contribute to an understanding of the responses of people to change.

Diffusion of innovation

Diffusion of innovation theories are social-psychological and sociological theories used to explain patterns of adoption of innovations, particularly technological innovations. Innovations are defined as 'ideas, practices or objects that are perceived as new. It matters little whether or not the idea is objectively new' (Rogers 1995, p. 11).

One theory of innovation diffusion was developed by Everett Rogers (1995), who argued that potential users evaluate an innovation in terms of its relative advantage, compatibility, ease of use, trialability, and visibility. An innovation that is perceived to be better than the idea it supersedes, and compatible with the existing values, experience, and needs of potential adopters, is more likely to be adopted. An innovation that is easy to understand and able to be experimented with will be adopted more rapidly, and the easier it is for individuals to see the results of an innovation, the more likely they are to adopt it. In the health environment, the range of professional groups may well result in different assessments of an innovation.

Organisational characteristics also influence the diffusion process. These are size, degree of centralisation of power and control, complexity of professional groups, the relative emphasis on rules and procedures, availability of uncommitted resources, and voluntary or involuntary adoption. Current thinking suggests an innovation may be successfully introduced into most environments if the particular characteristics of an organisation are matched with strategies to introduce the innovation.

Rogers sees opinion leaders as being an important element in the innovation diffusion process. He argues that most individuals evaluate an innovation not on the basis of scientific research by experts, but through the subjective evaluations of peers who have adopted the innovation. Opinion leaders may influence others to adopt an innovation. In conservative organisations, however, opinion leaders may influence others to reject an innovation.

Diffusion of innovation theory explains a process. The diffusion process is not always managed in the sense of being a planned, methodical process but if the innovation will generate significant changes in an organisation, it will generally be more successful if it is planned and managed.

Planned change

Organisations are evolving entities. There are times, however, when an organisation experiences quite rapid change. Without some planning and management, rapid change can be disruptive to the organisation and its members. In today's environment, rapid and dramatic change is occurring more frequently and information technology is increasingly involved in organisation change.

The field of change management focuses on understanding and enabling the change process. It is a significant area of study, which can only touched upon here. There are many resources that provide a more in-depth discussion of a range of management and change management concepts, including Martin et al. 2002.

Discussions of change management include theories that seek to understand and explain organisation change, and approaches and tools to facilitate successful management. It will come as no surprise that, since change management is located within the social sciences, there are many theories and strategies, with no single theory or strategy considered the 'right' approach. Current thinking is that planned change needs to be understood and tailored to fit the specific needs of an organisation within its cultural, economic, and political context.

Theories and strategies of change management are shaped by assumptions about an organisation and its members. One way of categorising these is as follows:

- *Empirical-rational*: assumes that people, once they realise that it is in their interests to do so, will accept change. Strategies within this category emphasise communication and rewards.
- *Normative-reductive*: adopts a cultural approach to understanding and managing change. A basic assumption is that people are social beings guided by cultural norms and values. Change management seeks to redefine existing norms and values.
- *Power-coercive*: assumes that people will essentially do what they are told, or can be made to do so. Strategies focus on authoritarian, top-down approaches and the use of sanctions for non-compliance.
- *Environmental-adaptive*: based on the assumption that, although people oppose change, they will adapt to new circumstances. Strategies within this category focus on 'building' a new organisation as people move from the old structures to the new ones.

While some assumptions and ideas may seem more attractive than others, all may be successful when used appropriately. Elements common to most theories include:

- the human factor, in that it is important to work with people who are involved in the change process
- the dynamic nature of change and its impact on all systems within the organisation
- embedding the change into the structures of the organisation
- the importance of communication
- change involving technology, which may involve a long learning curve, pointing to the need for incremental change.

Health enterprises with a traditional hierarchical structure are often slow to adopt information technology (Anderson 1997, Saranummi et al 2001, Tanriverdi & Iacono 1998), whereas the more teamwork-oriented organisation is more receptive to the introduction of information systems (Whetton 2002). Yet, traditional, hierarchical organisations do successfully implement changes, including the introduction of information systems, if strategies are planned to match the particular characteristics of the organisation.

A LITTLE SOCIAL SCIENCE

Theories from the social sciences contribute to the socio-technical focus of health informatics by facilitating an analysis of:

- the key players and their perspectives
- the impact of changes on various groups
- the meaning of information systems from user perspectives.

In Chapter 2 it was noted that health informatics draws upon positivist, interpretive, and critical methods for its scientific research. These represent different perspectives in the social world, and different ways to observe, measure, and understand that world. None represents the true or correct view of the world, but each offers insights and together they contribute to a more comprehensive understanding.

Positivist perspectives

Positivism is the fundamental approach of the scientific worldview, which dominated physical and social research throughout the nineteenth century and most of the twentieth century. This is the approach most people think of when they think of science and scientific methods. Its methodology involves observations, hypotheses, and the collection of data or empirical evidence according to clearly defined rules, procedures, and techniques. Positivism uses quantitative research methods, collecting and manipulating data through experiments, surveys, and statistics. The emphasis is on objectivity, logic, and rational explanation of observed phenomena. Computer science and biomedicine have extensively utilised the positivist approach.

An analysis of articles in the *Journal of Telemedicine and Telecare* (Brisbane, 2003) shows a range of papers written from a positivist perspective. Table 3.4 lists some papers, their focus and methodology.

Interpretive perspectives

From the 1960s onwards, there was an increasing argument that positivism did not adequately explain the social world. Critics of positivist methodologies argued that the social world is made up of humans who think and act. We cannot, therefore, adequately explain the social world without taking into account the thoughts of the participants in the social world.

Table 3.4 Positivist perspectives

Research/study	Focus/findings	Methodology
Organisational readiness for telemedicine: implications for success or failure. (Penny Jennet et al.)	Systematic assessment of organisational factors such as planning readiness, strategic plan, needs assessment and analysis, business plan	Data collection from structured interviews
Managing risk in telemedicine (Robert McCrosin)	Risk management	Analysis of incident reports; root cause analysis
Teleneurology by email (Dr Victor Patterson, Jenny Humphreys, and Richard Chua)	Safety, effectiveness, and efficiency of application	Data collection, analysis of response times, and outcomes
Low bandwidth physical rehabilitation for total knee replacement patients: preliminary results (Trevor Russel, Peter Buttrum, Richard Wootton and Gwendolen Hull)	Efficacy of outpatient program	Statistical analyses of physical activity measures

Source: *Journal of Telemedicine and Telecare*, 2003

Interpretive social science therefore seeks to understand how people interpret and respond to their social world and to learn what is relevant and meaningful from their perspective. Interpretive research also explores the way people create the roles and relationships that make up their social world. This perspective, then, can contribute to our understanding of the culture and structure of health organisations. It can also identify the attitudes and beliefs of groups and individuals towards health informatics programs and initiatives.

To gather this information, interpretive social scientists use qualitative methods such as participant observation, field research, and in-depth interviews.

An area of interest for interpretative research is usability. An application is not in itself usable or unusable. The attributes of the application will determine the usability for a particular user in a particular environment. Since usability is defined from the point of view of the users, interpretive research is the most appropriate approach to usability testing. Examples of research adopting an interpretive perspective are shown in Table 3.5.

Table 3.5 Interpretive perspectives

Research/study	Focus/findings	Methodology
Factors influencing the uptake of telehealth (Judi Walker and Sue Whetton 2003)	Diffusion of telehealth technology	Qualitative content analysis of interviews
Communicating via video-phone with elderly patients who have cognitive impairment (Stefan Savenstedt , K. Zingmark and P. O. Sandman 2003)	Satisfaction with method of service delivery; quality of service	Qualitative content analysis of interviews
Evaluation and health information systems—an interpretive study (Eva Klecun-Dabrowska and Tony Cornford 2001)	Evaluation as a situated activity requiring a more interpretive approach	Semi-structured interviews
Doctors' experience with handheld computers in clinical practice: qualitative study (Anne Scheck McAlearney, Sharon Schweikhart and Mitchell Medow 2004)	Explores doctors' subjective perceptions of the technology in the work environment	Focus groups

Source: *Journal of Telemedicine and Telecare*, 2003

Critical perspectives

Whereas the interpretive perspective looks at the interactions and perceptions of individuals and small groups, critical research seeks to understand the larger social structures and how they shape the social world. It is therefore concerned with power relations and how the more dominant views shape our worldview.

A primary aim of the perspective is to conduct research to critique existing social arrangements and frequently to actively seek to change these. Clearly, this is not a focus of health informatics. The insights gained from adopting a critical perspective, however, can undoubtedly contribute to our understanding of the social environment of health by identifying social, political, and cultural drivers and the voices behind these. This perspective utilises both quantitative and qualitative research methods.

Examples of critical research in health informatics are shown in Table 3.6.

Table 3.6 Critical perspectives

Research/study	Focus/findings	Methodology
Developing prison telemedicine systems: the Greek experience (George Anogianakis et al.)	Resistance to use; bureaucratic and labour problems Interview	Analysis of documentation
Diffusion of telecare in the Australian health care system (David Hailey and Bernie Crowe)	Relative influence of key players	Document analysis

Source: *Journal of Telemedicine and Telecare*, 2003

SUMMARY

As an applied discipline, health informatics has drawn on other disciplines for many of the concepts and theories it uses to develop an understanding of health information management within the health care environment. Concepts are terms used to represent ideas or processes. The knowledge base of a discipline is structured around the concepts used to encapsulate the key ideas. In health informatics, information is a fundamental concept since it encapsulates the field. The concept of a model is also fundamental. Models are used to analyse, manipulate, and modify data and information and the environment within which the information will be managed. Since health care deals with personal information, security and its component parts is also an integral concept. These concepts are supplemented by concepts from the social sciences, which enable the adoption of a socio-technical perspective.

Systems theory is used widely within the discipline of health informatics. Systems theory is based on the assumption that complex systems such as the human body, or a health care organisation, are greater than their component parts. Understanding a system therefore requires that it be studied as a whole, rather than studying each individual component. Health care systems and health informatics systems have people as component parts. People use values, attitudes, and experiences in their responses to situations. They are not always predictable. The utilisation of theories from other social science disciplines, including education, social psychology, and sociology will enhance the understanding of the behaviour of people in systems.

WWW LINKS

Privacy

OECD Privacy Principles <http://www.oecd.org/home>

National health privacy legislation

Australia <http://www.privacy.gov.au/health>
Canada <http://www.privcom.gc.ca>
New Zealand <http://www.privacy.org.nz/>
United Kingdom <http://www.informationcommissioner.gov.uk/>
USA <http://www.hhs.gov/ocr/hipaa/privacy.html>

CRITICAL THINKING

The executive management team of the typical health care system discussed in this chapter is intending to implement a system-wide intranet to disseminate information, including patient information, to staff.

1   Create a model of the health system in its environment.
2   How might an understanding of the culture and structure of the health system facilitate the change-management process required to move staff from a print-based system to the intranet?
3   Identify data, information, and knowledge that might be included on the intranet site.
4   How might learning theories facilitate the development of a usable intranet?
5   What conflicts can you see between the need to offer high quality health care and the need to protect personal information?

HEALTH INFORMATICS TOOLS, TECHNIQUES, AND APPLICATIONS

This second part of the book focuses on the tools and techniques used to manage health information. While these chapters explore the technology, the issues raised are predominantly those relating to the 'socio' rather than the technical aspects of health informatics. These include the influence of key player perspectives on the development of services and programs.

Chapter 4 reviews basic hardware, software, and networking technology, identifying a number of the core issues that recur throughout this part. These include the need to match systems to user requirements, the value of planning, standards, security and usability, roles, relationships, work processes, and routines.

Chapter 5 explores the concepts, structures, processes, and purposes of databases in the health care environment, while Chapter 6 focuses on health information systems. While this chapter introduces the general features of information systems, the focus is on the large health administration systems that have evolved over the last few decades. Issues around these **legacy systems** are discussed, along with other social and technical issues.

Chapter 7 explores the complex, dynamic, evolving e-health environment, Chapter 8 focuses on the electronic health record and Chapter 9 discusses developments in decision support systems in the health care environment.

CHAPTER 4

TOOLS: PROMISES AND PITFALLS

OVERVIEW

Health informatics is about the management of health information. Information and communications technology is increasingly the tool of choice for health information management. It is essential to have an understanding of these tools, their capabilities and limitations. This ensures that systems are able to perform the functions they are required to do. It also ensures consideration of the issues and challenges arising from the use of these tools in the health care environment. Attention to these issues and challenges will help to ensure that the applications and services created from the basic tools will be effective and efficient.

OBJECTIVES

At the completion of this chapter, you should be able to:
- describe the basic tools and components of health information and communications technology
- outline issues to be considered when using information and communications technology tools
- discuss issues and themes that underlie the success of health informatics in the health care environment.

CONCEPTS

Hardware	Wide area network
Software	Intranet
Networks	Internet
Local area network	Extranet

INTRODUCTION

The chapter begins by considering some current uses of information and communications technology in health care services. It identifies and discusses hardware, software, and networking tools, and identifies issues influencing their use. Since these basic tools combine to create health information systems and applications, the chapter, therefore, lays the foundation for the chapters that follow.

USING THE TOOLS

Blue skies or stormy weather

The complex health care environment, with its emphasis on consumer-centred service delivery, continuity of care across services, and movement of resources and services beyond the traditional hospital base, has put increasing pressure on traditional information management methods. The need to find new ways of structuring, managing, sharing, and using health care information has seen health services increasingly turn to information and communication technology tools. The use of these tools is leading to the emergence of new service delivery models. This is illustrated in Box 4.1.

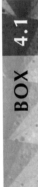

BOX 4.1

BLUE SKIES

It is 10.30 a.m. and Lei-Zi Daze has arrived for a consultation with Dr Azure Vault at the Blue Skies Community Health Centre. Lei-Zi suffers from a rare and intractable tropical disease, contracted while he was living in the Amazon. There have only been two cases of this illness treated in Australia in the last five years, but there is a well-managed treatment program in the USA, and they help to manage Lei-Zi as a remote patient, with Dr Vault as the local responsible clinician. Lei-Zi actively monitors his condition himself, accessing patient information and a support group through the website of the US centre. He enters results of self-administered blood tests and clinical observations into his online record. This record (on the Internet, requiring password access) automatically alerts Dr Vault when a result is entered that is outside the expected range. Lei-Zi's latest test results were unusual. Dr Vault had her system send an SMS message to Lei-Zi's mobile, asking him to ring. Lei-Zi called and made an appointment for a face-to-face consultation. Dr Vault accessed the online medical databases for the latest information about Lei-Zi's condition. Lei-Zi has also reviewed current information and he and Dr Vault explore treatment options together. The decisions are entered into Lei-Zi's online record, and will be reviewed by a specialist in the US centre when he starts work in a few hours. A prescription is generated and will be ready for Lei-Zi when he calls in at his usual pharmacy, while the relevant details of the consultation are automatically forwarded to the Health Insurance Commission, the Office of Public Health, and the state health department. Lei-Zi has given consent for these details to be communicated, and understands who will receive them, and why. He has also consented for the Centre to direct debit his bank account for the consultation.

Also at the Health Centre this morning are:

- **Dr Heesa Stork**, who is conducting the regular antenatal clinic via IP (Internet Protocol) videoconference to the seven remote communities serviced by the Centre. Dr Stork has online access to the latest test results and scans for each member of the group. These have been automatically uploaded from the specialist services in Global Metropolis, and the local diagnostic unit. The program began with six participants, but there were twenty-one at the last session.

- **The Centre Executive Committee** are videoconferencing with the Regional Executive Officer, based at Cloud Free Hospital in Sun City. They are discussing the next phase of the recently implemented Regional Patient Information System. This system has successfully integrated several administrative and financial legacy systems. The Committee is now looking to develop a regional electronic health record incorporating clinical information.

- **Diabetes specialist, Lynne Insuleyn,** who is considering the next phase of a successful online education program for community nurses. The web pages were designed to ensure the program was accessible regardless of the type of Internet connections nurses had. Lynne wants to talk to the development team about expanding the program for diabetes patients and the general community.

Blue Skies illustrates successful applications of:

- *E-health and telehealth*: Consumers in Blue Skies are accessing reliable, accredited, high quality websites to enable them to become more knowledgeable about health issues. They are also using e-health to access health and medical care not available locally. The designers of these programs and services are facilitating this by taking into account usability issues. The Blue Skies Community Health Centre demonstrates the versatility of telehealth in service provision to remote or isolated areas with its clinical, education, and administrative services.

- *Integrated information systems*: The Blue Skies–Cloud Free Regional Patient Information System demonstrates the potential for more effective and efficient administration through the integration of health information systems.

- *Electronic health records*: Blue Skies Community Health Centre, in collaboration with regional health services, is developing a secure online patient records system, which will enable health professionals in geographically diverse locations to access essential patient information.
- *Evidence-based practice*: Traditionally, health professionals relied on their professional knowledge, experience, and common sense for clinical practice and for evaluating new treatments and diagnoses. Rare or unusual problems were solved by consulting text books or asking colleagues. Doctor Vault uses the contemporary approach of electronic databases and email to maintain her knowledge base and ensure high quality health care.

Unfortunately, Blue Skies is in 'Don't You Wish' land, where everything works according to plan. In the real world, health informatics and other professionals can expect problems to arise as new information management strategies and systems are planned, developed, and implemented. Box 4.2 illustrates a number of the issues they can expect to confront.

BOX 4.2

STORMY WEATHER

At the Cloudy Village Community Health Centre, Mary Tee has arrived for her appointment with Dr Ima Luddite. Mary has HIV, which she normally manages via a support group on the Internet. She tries to discuss the information she gains from this group with Dr Luddite, who is resentful of Mary's 'meddling'. Last time Mary logged into the group, her information was harvested by the overseas pharmaceutical company that funds the site anonymously. The company continues to send Mary unsolicited advice and offers to sell her cut-price drugs. In spite of her reservations, she feels more comfortable dealing with the Internet site than with her grumpy GP. She purchased her last month's drugs online, but the ones she received were a little different from those she usually takes, and that appears to have exacerbated her illness.

Dr Luddite thinks the Internet is a fad. To gain the latest information on treatments and diagnoses she relies on printed journals, when she has time to read them, and discussions with colleagues on her golf day. She has never heard of the drugs Mary has been taking. Dr Luddite wrote a prescription for a drug she has been prescribing for HIV for a year or two now. The prescription was automatically transmitted to the local pharmacy. Unfortunately Mary's record was left displayed on the pharmacy screen where the local busybody read it. Mary's details were also automatically forwarded to the Health Insurance Commission, the Office of Public Health, and the state health department. Mary had signed a consent form for this. Unfortunately an employee at the state health department was running a business on the side selling medical information to insurance companies and employers. Mary lost her job and has had her life insurance policy cancelled for no stated reason.

Also at the Health Centre were:

- **Dr Heesa Stork**, who was to conduct the regular antenatal clinic via videoconference to the three remote communities serviced by the Centre. The clinic was implemented because the Clinical Team Leader thought it would be a good idea to have a 'telemedicine presence'. Funding was allocated for the establishment of the program, but there is very little available for maintenance, call costs, support, or upgrades. This is not working well, since the low bandwidth ISDN connection is not sufficient and the quality of the transmission is extremely poor (when the connection can be made). Dr Stork is not happy. She has to leave her consulting room to conduct the clinic, and privacy is not guaranteed in the multi-purpose room where the video-conferencing equipment is located.

- **The Centre Executive Committee**, which is holding a videoconference meeting with the Executive Officer of the region, based at Thunder Box Hospital in Storm City. They are discussing difficulties with the recently installed Regional Patient Information System. Due to incompatibility issues, only two of the five systems have been integrated so far. Staff are having difficulty using the systems. They require significant changes in their work routines and they resent these being 'imposed from above'. The project is experiencing a significant cost and time overrun.

- **Diabetes specialist**, Lynne Insuleyn, who is trying to salvage an online education program for community nurses. The program is not being used because it is too difficult to navigate, the images take too long to download, and the help files are written in techno-jargon. Many users are still accessing the site using dial-up modems.

Cloudy Village illustrates some of the issues needing to be addressed when developing and implementing systems and programs. These include:

- *Technical issues*: It is important that user needs are clearly identified, and are supported by the technology, rather than imposing a technical solution that forces inappropriate changes in work patterns. The systems in Cloudy Village do not have the hardware, software, and networking capabilities to meet user needs. The consequences of this are seen in the slow, unreliable, poor quality systems and, in the case of the patient information system, incompatible systems. These programs also highlight problems that can arise from a lack of a clear plan about what is required, what is achievable, and what resources are necessary. An additional issue is the rapid evolution of technology, which sees many systems outdated in a very short space of time. If these systems are updated, organisations often find that applications or other parts of the system also require upgrading. Thus we have a situation not dissimilar to that discussed in Chapter 1, where expectations for the latest technology are outstripping the ability or willingness of organisations to pay.

- *Security*: Although computer security techniques help to maintain the confidentiality, integrity, and availability of the resources maintained by a computer system, Cloudy Village overlooked the fact that technical solutions provide only half of the answer. The harvesting of information from websites, inappropriate location and display of personal information, and illegitimate use of information by individuals with legitimate access, point to the other half of the problem—the behaviour of systems users. Business rules, security policies, and adequate training of both staff and consumers are just as important in preventing the misuse of information of health systems as are security techniques.

- *Usability issues*: We know that a significant factor in the acceptance or rejection of any health system or application by its users is the system's usability. Both the diabetes education program and the integrated patient information systems at Cloudy Village appear to be victims of insufficient attention paid to usability.

- *Professional and cultural issues*: The relationship between Dr Luddite and Mary Tee points to issues around changing professional and consumer relationships. While this particular example may appear to be outside the influence of the health informatics professional, we should consider strategies to facilitate the adoption of these emerging models of interaction. The workflow issues are clearly within the scope of planning and implementation activities.

As with Blue Skies, this illustration is necessarily simplified. Real life is much more complex. The example does, however, point to the need to understand the tools of health informatics. This chapter begins by focusing on the hardware, software, and networks tools that are the foundation of databases, information systems, electronic records, and e-health programs.

KNOWING THE TOOLS

The first step to ensuring that information and communication technologies will enable rather than inhibit or complicate services is understanding the tools that are used. We need to be clear about what technologies are available and what they are capable of doing. This will enable us to work more effectively with computer and other specialists to choose the configurations that best suit the needs of each health care environment.

Stand alone computers

When it was finished, the ENIAC filled an entire room, weighed thirty tons, and consumed two hundred kilowatts of power. It generated so much heat that it had to be placed in one of the few rooms at the University with a forced air-cooling system. Vacuum tubes, over 19 000 of them, were the principal elements in the computer's circuitry (Richey 2004).

One of the earliest computers, developed in the USA in the 1940s, was the Electronic Numerical Integrator and Computer (ENIAC). ENIAC was controlled by a set of external switches and dials. The machine was completed in 1945.

Australia was not far behind. In 1947, a research group at the Radiophysics Laboratory of the Council for Scientific and Industrial Research began work on an Australian computer. When it first ran in late 1949, CSIR Mk1 became the fifth electronic stored program computer in the world.

We have come a long way since ENIAC. Computers have been getting faster, smaller, and more mobile, and their ability to manipulate and store information has been increasing exponentially since they first emerged into the commercial and business environment during the 1960s. Table 4.1 shows the main categories of computers in use today.

Table 4.1 Categories of computer

Category	Description
Embedded systems programming computer	A computer that is embedded in something and does not support direct human interaction but nevertheless meets all the other criteria of a microcomputer. Appliances with a digital interface, such as microwave ovens and VCRs, utilise embedded systems.
Microcomputer	A standard personal computer.
Workstation	A more powerful personal computer for special applications. The term is sometimes used to mean an individual personal computer hooked up to a mainframe computer.
Minicomputer	A computer of a size intermediate between a microcomputer and a mainframe.
Point of service	Portable computers, handheld, and sometimes wireless (cellular) devices, which are used to gather data at multiple locations and transmit it to the information system.
Cluster	Often several microcomputers or larger computers that share a workload and back each other up.
Mainframe or mainframe computer	Now usually referred to by its manufacturers as a 'large server'.
Supercomputer	A very large server, sometimes including a system of computers using parallel processing.
Parallel processing system	A system of interconnected computers that work on the same application together, sharing tasks that can be performed.

Health care environments vary widely and the attributes of these different computers make them more suitable in one context than in another. We need to ensure that the information and communications technologies (ICTs) we introduce are indeed the most appropriate for that environment. An example: 'wireless devices were ideal for certain clinical areas, while other departments such as critical and long-term care were best suited to bedside PCs, or point-of-care technology' (Pooley 2002, p. 19).

Given the rapid rate of technology development, the issue of suitability requires constant review. Modifications and enhancements may see inappropriate systems evolving to become the best fit and vice versa.

Computers as systems

Computers are systems. They consist of input devices, processing devices, storage devices, and output devices. These combine and interact with each other to perform functions the individual components are unable to do. As this is a computer system, data is the input entered into the system from the environment. It is processed, and stored until needed, at which time it then becomes output. Table 4.2 shows the devices used to input, process, store, and output data in a computer system.

Table 4.2 Devices used to input, process, store, and output data in a computer system

Function	Device
Input	Keyboard, mouse, digital camera, monitor, scanner, video digitiser, microphone, joy stick, light pen, modem.
Processing	The Central Processing Unit (CPU) transforms the data. The CPU consists of electrical circuits, which carry out instructions from the software and the operating system. The more circuits there are in the CPU, the faster the computer. The speed is measured in megahertz (MHz), or millions of cycles per second. The higher the megahertz, the faster the computer.
Storage	Hard disk, floppy disk, CD ROM, DVD, memory stick, RAM, smart card, magnetic stripe.
Output	Monitor, liquid crystal displays (LCDs), speakers, printer, modem.

The hard drive, which is part of the computer box, and portable devices such as floppy disks, CD ROMs, and memory sticks, are long-term data storage devices. The portable devices are used to store information away from the computer and to transport information from one location to another.

Random access memory (RAM) is the short-term working memory. Any current work is stored in the RAM. It will not go into the long-term storage until it is saved. RAM never runs out of memory. It keeps operating, but as it stores more and more work in progress, it operates much more slowly than you may want it to. If you close an application, turn off the computer, or there is a power failure before you save work, it will be lost. The size of the RAM is an important factor in the performance of a computer. Insufficient RAM will result in a very slow computer.

Memory is measured in bytes. Memory size is usually described as being in kilobytes, megabytes, gigabytes, and terabytes. Very large computers have memories measured as petabytes, while supercomputers may have memories measured in exabytes.

Files

Files are used to store data and information in a computer. Although there are several different types of files, computers mainly deal with executable files and data files. Executable files contain the instructions the computer needs to perform particular tasks. Every application begins with an executable file. Without executable files a computer will not run. Data files generally contain data rather than instructions. In recent years, however, the distinction between data files and executable files has blurred considerably. Fairly simple word processor and spreadsheet files can now include 'macros' and small segments of programming code that enable quite complex and sophisticated functions. Web pages often include components such as ActiveX and Java code, which are able to run automatically as small programs on the local computer. Data files may contain any mix of pictures, text, sounds, movies, music, or numbers. File types can usually be identified by their file extension. Some examples are shown in Table 4.3. You should note that some file extensions are generic, while others refer to specific software. For example, the file extension .pdf refers specifically to Adobe Acrobat files.

Table 4.3 Types of files

File type	Extension
Executable files	.exe
	.dll
Data files	
Text files	.txt .doc
Database files	.db .mdb .xml .fpt
Spreadsheet	.wks .xls
Sound	.aiff .wav .mp3 .au
Graphics	.bmp .pcx .jpg .gif
Animation, video	.flc .avi .mpg .js
Web documents	.html .htm .asp

To open a file, the computer usually needs a program that stores that type of data file. A word processing program, for example, would not usually be able to open a .jpg file, but may be able to do so with extra software components such as 'translators' or 'filters'. In a recent development, program developers are using the web page file format as the standard way to store data. Any browser on any computer can read standard html files, although some more complicated html files may only display correctly in a particular browser. This makes it easy to transfer between computers.

Software for stand alone computers

Without *software*, a computer is just a useless gadget. Software sets the tasks for the computer to perform, then tells the computer how to go about performing the tasks.

There is a huge range of software. Table 4.4 lists the most common categories.

Table 4.4 Computer software

Software	Purpose
Operating systems	The operating system controls everything the computer does. It is used by the system to open the other programs. The most well-known operating systems today are Microsoft Windows, used for PCs; Mac OS, used for Macintosh computers; and UNIX, which can be used by both.
Word processing applications	Word processing software allows you to create and store a wide range of documents in electronic files in your computer, or on your organisation's server. Electronic files can easily be edited, formatted, and integrated with other types of applications, such as a spreadsheet or a database management program.
Presentation software	Multimedia presentation software with the capability to incorporate text, graphics, sound, animation, and video into a file for presentation.
Database applications	These are a key tool for health informatics. A database is a collection of data or information. The database management system (DBMS) is a program used to create, maintain, and work with databases. The DBMS ensures data integrity (ensuring accessibility and consistency in organisation of data) and security (ensuring that only those with access privileges can access the data).
Spreadsheets	Spreadsheets are also used to store, organise, and manipulate data. Spreadsheets deal with numbers and perform a wide range of mathematical, financial, and statistical functions. Spreadsheets are used to organise data, compute and summarise information, model scenarios, generate reports, and produce graphs or charts. They are excellent for numerical analyses.
Entertainment software	Extremely popular, frustrating, time-consuming, but enjoyable software.

COMPUTER PLATFORMS

Platforms are a way of grouping computers of similar design. With desktop computers, for example, Macintosh (Mac) computers are one platform, while PCs running the Microsoft Windows operating system are another. When people talk about computers being compatible, they generally mean that they can use the same software and peripheral devices. Older Macs and PCs are generally incompatible. Later versions of Macs are able to use many of the applications designed for PCs. These applications are called multi-platform. Compatibility applies to both software and peripheral devices.

Networked computers

Today, very few computers are stand-alone systems. The vast majority are linked to other computers via some form of network. There are basically two kinds of networks. The first is the local area network (LAN), which links computers located within one organisation or geographical area. LANs usually have restricted access. A LAN can be connected to other LANs to form a wide area network (WAN). Wide area networks link geographically distributed computers and networks together. The Internet is the best known WAN. Another form of WAN is an extranet, which is a private network used to enable business organisations to share data and information.

Local area networks

Computers in a LAN can be connected via fixed or wireless networks. Traditional fixed networks consist of six components:

- *Computers*: Computers include personal computers, or workstations, and servers. There are basically two configurations used for networks. These are client–server and peer-to-peer networks. In client–server networks, one or more computers control and provide access to shared resources. In peer-to-peer networks, each computer has exactly the same function and rights as all the others.
- *Protocols*: Protocols define the rules and signals that computers on the network use to format and communicate data. There are a number of different protocols that can be used. Computers in a network must support the appropriate protocols if they are to communicate with other computers.
- *Network interface card*: A network interface card is a circuit board that sends data from the workstation out over the network and collects data from the network for the workstation. Each device in the network must have a network card. Different networks use different types of network interface cards.
- *Network cables*: Computer networks are generally connected via some kind of cable. Today, wireless networks are increasingly common. In wireless networks, specialised transmitters may replace some or all of the functions of network interface cards, hubs, switches, routers, and gateways, making network cables unnecessary.
- *Hubs or switches, routers or gateways*: these perform traffic control. The devices basically read the destination address on the packets of information being sent by a computer and then forward it to the appropriate destination.

- *Service devices*: Network devices include printers, and data services, which provide additional support to the network.

Wide area networks—the Internet

The Internet has evolved over the past thirty years from an initial experiment with four computers into the current huge information network that connects millions of micro-computers, mainframes, and supercomputers.

As with many information communications technologies, the Internet had its beginnings with the military. During the 1960s, the USA was involved in a number of conflicts or potential conflict situations. The military argued that there was a need for a secure (and bomb proof) communications system that would allow military person-nel to communicate with each other in the event of war. In response to this, the US Defence Advance Research Projects Administration (DARPA) commissioned a study on computer-to-computer communication technologies. The project was referred to as Advanced Research Projects Agency Net (ARPANET) and worked on the theory that if one part of a system network failed (in terms of the Cold War, a city might be knocked out by a nuclear strike) then the message would be rerouted via another path. The rerouting would continue until the message reached the intended recipient. This meant that if one computer was destroyed, communication would continue because the network offered other paths.

As shown in Figure 4.1, this is how the Internet works today. Messages are routed via other computers and no direct connection is necessary between the sender and the receiver. The actual path taken is determined at the time of communication, and can vary during transmission. This will be decided according to the traffic on the Internet.

Figure 4.1 How the Internet works

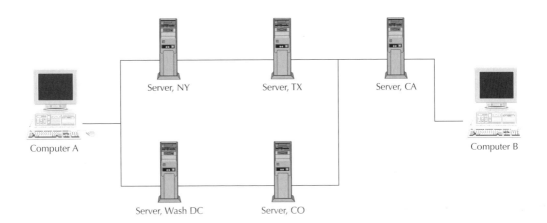

Source: from Beginners Central 1998

The link between Computer A and Computer B can take several paths. It might travel hundreds, even thousands of miles out of the way to reach the other computer. Fortunately, it will (usually) get there.

Computers are connected to the Internet via hosts. Hosts are any device having a permanent connection to the Internet. There are several ways to connect to the Internet. Table 4.5 lists the main methods.

Table 4.5 Network connection options

Connection type	Description	Speed
Dial-up modem	The most common method of connection. Modems use the telephone line.	Modems range in speed from 14 kilobits per second (Kbps) to 56 Kbps and are the slowest connections. It may be difficult to download websites with animation, or lots of graphics.
ISDN	ISDN stands for Integrated Services Digital Network. It operates over standard telephone wires and fibre optic circuits. ISDN is used by larger organisations.	Speeds are around 128 Kbps.
ADSL Broadband	ADSL stands for Asymmetric Digital Subscriber Line and is currently one of the fastest internet connections available. ADSL also operates over standard phone lines.	Broadband, at 1000 Kbps, is much faster than dial-up modem.
Satellite	A satellite connection converts digital signals to radio waves, sending information via satellite. It is available almost anywhere, which makes it very promising, although expensive, for rural areas.	Satellite connections have been measured at between 200 and 1350 Kbps.
Wireless	The newest Internet technology, this form of connection uses either radio frequency or an infra-red port connection. It does not need cables or wires. Large businesses and hospitals are beginning to use wireless for inventory, file sharing, business records, and email.	Wireless connections can access the Internet at a speed of 11 Mbps.

The type of Internet connection will have a significant impact on the efficiency with which different types of information can be uploaded or downloaded. At the same time, the type of connection that is possible will depend on the services available in the region/location, or within a particular organisation. The health informatics professional needs to be aware that these technical options matter, since they have an impact on the use of information. The practicalities of implementation are, however, the focus of IT/network professionals.

Internet services

People tend to think of the Internet in terms of logging on, searching or browsing, and viewing web pages, but there are a number of other services available. Table 4.6 outlines these.

MANAGING THE TOOLS

By combining the insights gained from Blue Skies and Cloudy Village with an understanding of the characteristics of the basic hardware, software, and networking tools, we can identify a number of issues and themes that underlie the success of health informatics in the health care environment.

Matching technology to user requirements

Health services and health professionals have been consistently reluctant to adopt health informatics applications. If you explore the reasons for this, you may find that the applications have been frequently perceived as:

- *Not suitable or appropriate for the particular requirements*: We saw, in Cloudy Village, that the technology was not appropriate for the type of service it was being used for. The use of graphics and animation on a website primarily accessed via dial-up modem is an example of this.
- *Interrupting the usual workflow*: We also saw this in Cloudy Village, where staff resisted the regional patient information system because it was impacting on their work routines.
- *Difficult to use*: Poorly designed applications, again as in the case of the Cloudy Village diabetes education web page and regional patient information system, will be resisted.

Failure to match the technology to user requirements is often the result of inadequate thought and planning.

Planning

Health informatics applications are often imposed on services by senior decision makers. Sometimes they are acquired because vendors persuade unsuspecting senior clinicians of their value, because they seemed like a good idea at the time, because

Table 4.6 Internet services

Internet service	Description
World Wide Web	The World Wide Web is that part of the Internet where you view 'Internet sites' using your browser. Internet Explorer and Netscape are examples of browsers. You can think of the WWW as a library, with the millions of sites representing books. However, unlike a library, the books (websites) are not gathered in one place. The websites are located in millions of computers worldwide. As a result, the physical location becomes irrelevant. You can access materials anywhere in the world instantly.

When you 'search the Web', you are not searching it directly. Since web pages are stored on computers all over the world, your computer could not find or go to them all directly. What you do is access one of several intermediate databases, which contain selections of web pages. These are search engines. They are organised to allow you to find other web pages. Search engines provide hypertext links to other pages (URLs). |
Email	Email, or electronic mail, is probably the most frequently used feature of the Internet. It is simply correspondence conducted via a computer network. At its most simple, email can be used to send text messages, but it can also be used to send word processed documents, images, video clips, and linked web addresses. The ability to subscribe to mailing lists means that email can be a useful information-retrieval tool, discussion forum, and general group communication medium.
File transfer protocol	Computers work with data and programs. An integral part of the Internet is the transfer of the data and programs from one computer to another. File transfer protocol (FTP) is the set of rules that allows files on the Internet to be moved from one location to another. The FTP allows the user to download software, upload his or her own web pages, and transfer information between home and work machines.
Telnet	Telnet is a service that allows you to connect to remote computers on the Internet and use them in the same way as you would if you were sitting in front of them. Unlike the Web, Telnet does not support a graphical user interface. This means that the user needs to remember several keystroke commands, such as hitting the Ctrl and X keys simultaneously to end a Telnet session.

Newsgroups	Also known as USENET, newsgroups are discussion areas where people post messages to the group. It is the Internet equivalent of a bulletin board. Some groups are moderated while others are essentially a free for all. There are many health- and medicine-oriented newsgroups on the Internet.
Internet relay chat	Internet relay chat (IRC) is a 'real time' version of a newsgroup. It is synchronous communication. People involved in the discussion are online at the same time. At any one time, there are thousands of chat lines running simultaneously.

funding was available, or because project sponsors were particularly interested in the application. Any of these reasons can result in inappropriate systems. There are several examples of this in Cloudy Village. A more effective approach, as we saw in Blue Skies, is to ensure that each project contributes to the overall strategic goals of the organisation, and to plan for implementation in a way that will maximise effectiveness and minimise disruption. There are several phases in the management of a project.

Business case

It is usual to document the costs, benefits, and risks inherent in a project in a formal business case. This business case will allow those who control spending to assess whether the proposed project is a good fit for the organisation's strategic directions, and whether it represents a good use of the organisation's resources.

Project definition

Defining the project involves identifying the problem, and providing a clear description of the scope of the proposed solution (which may, or may not, be technology) in the context of the organisation's overall direction. Blue Skies might have, as part of its strategic goal, promotion of professional education for staff. It may have identified that rural and remote nurses are not receiving enough professional education. The problem is the provision of timely information to rural and remote nurses. The solution (tested against other options) is the development of an information website they can view from their home computer or local public facilities. Once the problem has been identified, the *outputs* of the project (those things that will be produced and implemented) and the intended *outcomes* (the resulting positive changes in the organisation and its services) are clearly described. These descriptions of outputs and outcomes help to identify the limits of the project. Project definition also involves listing benefits to key stakeholders, which may include the funding body, local health care providers, and the organisation itself, and outlining the human, material, and the financial resources required. The project definition phase is critical, since once the decision is made to proceed, the documentation produced in this phase will serve as a blueprint for the entire project.

Project planning

Project planning produces the project plan. Yet this is a living document. It evolves and changes as the project progresses. The project leader may develop a first draft project plan, but this will be reviewed, revised, and expanded when the full project team is assembled. It may then be revised again after consultations with key stakeholders, or after a review of available resources or at any other time through the life of the project. Project planning is also a participative process involving key stakeholders and team members.

Project control and monitoring

Most projects of a significant size will be implemented by a project team, with overall direction provided by a steering committee. The steering committee should ensure that the project stays within the original scope, that appropriate resources are provided, and that impediments to the project from within the organisation are managed. The development of most health informatics projects is an iterative process, involving constant evaluation and review. As each stage is completed, the project team evaluates both the outcome of that phase, and the way it was achieved. If modifications to the plan are required, they are recommended to the steering committee for approval. The project team (managed by the project manager) will organise and perform the work of the project, and will regularly report on the progress to the steering committee and the stakeholders. Unfortunately, many projects are not adequately evaluated during the development of a project.

Project completion and review

Strategies to evaluate the success of the final project must also be devised. Once the outputs have been delivered, it is necessary to ensure that the intended outcomes (business benefits) are realised. This is usually the responsibility of those who manage the staff using the new system. Clear objectives will be invaluable here, and will be strongly guided by the intended outputs and outcomes established during project definition. Evaluation strategies can range from collecting numerical data, such as the number of site visits, to the collection of more qualitative data, such as feedback from consumers or users. The end of project evaluation should be an extension of the evaluation conducted throughout the lifecycle of the project. Unfortunately it is often the case that evaluation occurs only on completion of the project.

The LASCAD project provides a useful case study for thinking about this planning process. Although this event occurred over a decade ago, many of the mistakes continue to be made. Box 4.3 summarises the LASCAD experience.

Compatibility

Early health care applications were often located in individual machines or, if networked, were confined to single departments. Individual departments often had the responsibility of selecting their own systems, and this was frequently done in isolation and without consultation with other departments. As a result, many organisations

BOX 4.3

LONDON AMBULANCE SERVICE COMPUTER AIDED DESPATCH (LASCAD) SYSTEM

Major objective

The primary goal of the LASCAD system was to automate many of the human-intensive processes of manual despatch systems associated with ambulance services in the United Kingdom.

The process

British Telecom was to route all 999 medical emergency calls to London Ambulance Service headquarters. Receivers would record the details of the patient and transmit the information over a local area network to an allocator. The system would pinpoint the patient's location on a map display. Continuous monitoring of the location of every ambulance via radio messages transmitted by each vehicle every 13 seconds, would enable the system to determine the ambulance nearest to the patient.

Components included a tracking system, communications system, a database, and a map-based display interface. It was an event-based system, using a rule-based approach in interaction with the geographical information system (GIS). It ran on a series of network PCs and file servers.

The breakdown

The system began operation on 26 October 1992. After two days, response time began to slow down, until it finally locked up altogether on 4 November. The following are comments from subsequent reviews and discussion about the project.

The business case was based on the high-risk assumption that the system would be capable of performing a near-perfect provision of information on vehicle location and crew/vehicle status. The policy of the NHS was that contracts should generally be awarded to the lowest tender. The project team misled the Ambulance Board over the level of experience of the contractors. The contract for the supply of software was awarded to a company with no previous experience building despatch systems for ambulance services. The detailed nature of the specification documents for the LASCAD project limited the ability for flexibility during the project planning and implementation stages. The specifications were prescriptive, with a high degree of precision on the way in which the system was intended to operate, allowing little scope for additional ideas to be incorporated. Senior management adopted an overambitious project timetable. Project management was inadequate.

The lack of iterative planning resulted in limited process evaluation as the project evolved. The form of the system was a poor fit with the structure of the ambulance service, impacting significantly on the way in which staff carried out their jobs. Yet there was little or no involvement of ambulance crews in the planning process

The system had significant usability issues. Software was incomplete and unstable: the emergency back-up system remained untested. Training was incomplete and inconsistent.

today contain a number of different, often incompatible, applications. As a further complication, parts of many of these systems are still paper based. This approach has created information silos—each system collects and processes its own data and information.

As was seen in Cloudy Village, silo systems are a barrier to increased information sharing, since they are locked within one system, department, or organisation and are not available to other parts of the organisation or service. This is compounded by the many different systems and applications used.

Standards are seen as a means of overcoming the problem of incompatibility. Health informatics standards are widely accepted rules or specifications that enable health professionals to collect, store, and share health-related data, information, and knowledge in an electronic format. You will note that we do not use the term *universal* when referring to standards as there are a number of groups and organisations involved in the development of standards that enjoy varying degrees of acceptance and compliance. This is not a new situation. The world has operated on two standards for weights and measures for many decades. Standards for health informatics include vocabularies, structure and content, messaging, and **security standards**. Table 4.7 summarises these standards. They are explored in detail in Chapters 5–8.

Security

As was discussed in Chapter 3, health care services are obligated to implement security measures that keep health data and information accurate, current, safely stored, and available only for the purposes specified. Well-designed systems will include security measures as a matter of course and will incorporate standards to protect data and information from unauthorised or inadvertent access, or the disclosure of information. Yet security ultimately relies on people. As we saw in Cloudy Village, security measures were unable to prevent inappropriate display of information, unauthorised harvesting of data left on a website, or illegal use of data by an individual with authorised access. Box 4.4 is another example of possible security problems.

Workflows and work routines

Health information systems impact on the culture and structure of health care organisations. New technologies often disrupt traditional work routines, workflow, and work relationships. The location of equipment, the need to consult with others, and the protocols involved may all have an impact on workflow and routines. As we saw in Cloudy Village, the failure to minimise these disruptions may well result in resistance to systems. Tanriverdi and Iacono (1999) found that in the 'real' world the introduction of telemedicine often required changes to traditional workflows. Lack of attention to how the technology would integrate into existing organisational workflows impacted strongly on the extent to which it was accepted.

Table 4.7 Standards

Standard	Purpose
Vocabularies	Vocabulary standards apply particularly to clinical databases and information systems. Vocabularies provide guidelines for descriptive terms to facilitate understanding and accurate interpretation of clinical information.
Structure and content	Content standards aim to provide a clear description of the data elements to be included in databases. This includes establishing essential data elements, such as identifier, name, and location, and standardising data structures such as field length, data type, and acceptable data content for various fields.
Messaging	Health information is held in a range of formats in different systems. **Messaging standards** enable these disparate data sources to be shared between systems by establishing a format and a sequence for data transmission.
Security	These are standards to protect data from unauthorised or inadvertent access or disclosure of information.

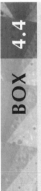

SECURITY

Monika Rola (2003) describes the privacy risks faced by general practitioners as they adopt information technology. Rola observes that even as their offices become automated, doctors remain naive as to what they should be doing to protect the sensitive data they hold. She also suggests that not many family physicians understand that their firewall, even if they have one installed, can have holes. As an example of the potential problems, Rola describes a GP office that gave a computer vendor access to its entire system via dial-up modem in case repairs were ever needed. When the vendor was asked if his employees could simply dial in and see the whole system, he answered 'Yes' and stated that they needed this access in order to do their jobs.

These issues will need to be dealt with in most health informatics projects. Different issues will be more significant in different environments, and different aspects of each issue will require attention in different applications.

SUMMARY

Effective management of health information is facilitated by an understanding of the tools used. Information and communications technology is increasingly the tool of choice for health information management. Effectively designed applications and services using these tools can contribute to more effective and more efficient health care, while poorly designed applications and services will create issues for users. Therefore, we need to be clear about what technologies are available and what they are capable of doing.

Computers, a fundamental tool, can be viewed as systems comprising input, processing, and output devices. Computer systems come in a variety of shapes and sizes, ranging from the standard microcomputer used by individuals to the very large mainframes and supercomputers used by large organisations. The different types of computer systems are suited to different environments and functions.

Today, very few computers operate as stand-alone systems. Most are networked. Networks are basically local area networks (LANs), located within one organisation or geographical area, or global networks linking hundreds or thousands (or millions in the case of the Internet) of geographically distributed machines. Connecting to global networks can be made via dial-up modem, ISDN, ADSL, satellite, or wireless.

Traditional fixed (cable connected) networks consist of computers, protocols to enable the formatting and communication of data, network interface cards, cables down which data is sent, and hubs, switches, or routers to control traffic on the network. In wireless networks, cables are redundant and transmitters replace some of the functions performed by network interface cards, hubs, and switches.

The Internet, the most widely used global network, offers a range of services, the most common of which are the World Wide Web, email, newsgroups, and Internet relay chat.

If these tools are to be used effectively, the technology must be matched to user requirements. This means that the technology must be appropriate for the intended purpose, be easy to use and have minimal impact on significant workflows and processes.

Planning is the key to achieving this. Planning ensures that the focus is on the problem or issue to be resolved, rather than on the technology to be used, that the proposed solution will meet the requirements of all key players, and that adequate attention will be paid to security, compatibility with existing systems, and usability.

WWW LINKS

Hardware, software, and networks

Geekgirl's plain English computing <http://www.geekgirls.com>

Computer Hope.com <http://www.computerhope.com/more.htm>

London Ambulance Service Computer Aided Despatch (LASCAD): Case study <http://www.scit. wlv.ac.uk/~cm1995/cbr/cases/case12/12.HTM>

CRITICAL THINKING

Use the planning steps discussed in the chapter to explore the problems of Cloudy Village. Consider the following issues.

1 Technical issues: identify the needs of various user groups, the technical and other limitations, and the steps required to overcome existing problems.

2 Security: distinguish between technical and human issues, identifying requirements for managing each of these.

3 Usability: what are the issues and how might they be avoided in the future?

4 Professional and cultural issues: how are the systems impacting on professional and cultural aspects of the Centre? What steps can be taken to minimise this on future projects?

CHAPTER 5

DOING DATABASES

OVERVIEW

Databases are a basic tool for health information management. Health and medical services are information dependent. Without access to accurate and timely information health professionals would not be able to offer high quality, efficient health care. In our **information society** the amount of data and information being generated has increased dramatically, making manual collection, organisation, and retrieval ever more cumbersome and time consuming. Electronic databases are increasingly becoming an essential tool for the collection and management of health data.

Databases have applications in clinical, research, education, and management areas. The increasing focus on evidence-based practice will see an increasing use of databases.

OBJECTIVES

After completing this chapter, you should be able to:
- distinguish between database structures
- discuss issues around legacy database systems in the health care environment
- outline steps for planning and implementing a health database
- discuss security and usability issues as they relate to health databases.

INTRODUCTION

There is an ever-increasing amount of information being collected and used by health and medical professionals today. In this information-intensive environment, data and information are being utilised in clinical, education, research, and administrative settings. As the volume of data and information being generated increases, databases and database management systems are becoming ever more important in assisting health professionals to collect, manage, maintain, and access the material.

Database development is a specialised field, requiring specific technical skills and knowledge. Designers of database systems are focused on the efficient use of computer memory, the design of systems that ensure the rapid retrieval of data, and on the safety and security of stored data.

Database design is a process that anyone can participate in. Potential users of databases should most certainly be involved in the design and development process. It will assist database designers to view the database from the end-user perspective and pay attention to usability and other user concerns. This will help to ensure that databases make the required information available in the right form to the right people in a usable manner.

The purpose of this chapter is to develop an understanding of the concepts and processes of database design and operation. It begins by discussing some types of databases and their uses. This includes a brief overview of database management systems and database architecture. This is followed by a general discussion of how a relational database might be planned, developed, and implemented. The final section reviews aspects of the finished database that will impact on its effectiveness and efficiency.

USING DATABASES

Databases are endemic in health information management. Both administrative and clinical health information systems incorporate at least one, and usually several, databases.

What are we talking about?

A database is an organised collection of related data. While a database may be manual, as with the data stored in the filing cabinet, or electronic, as with the data stored in a computer, the key characteristics of databases are that the data is organised systematically, enabling efficient retrieval, and that the data is related.

Repositories and information management

Some databases function as electronic *repositories of information*. They store vast quantities of data that can be searched for relevant information. Frequently such databases can be accessed through libraries, government agencies, professional organisations, and the Internet. The bodies that develop, update, and administer these databases determine who can access the information. Some have free public access, whereas others charge fees and/or limit access to specific groups of users. These databases are very much 'look but don't touch'. Authorised users can use search techniques to view, save, and print information, but cannot amend the information within the database. **Medline**, CHID Online (US Department of Health), and Omni (UK) are examples of health-related information repositories.

Other databases function as *information management tools*. Organisations or individuals create databases to store, sort and manipulate information to suit certain needs. This approach is 'hands on'. The information is usually specific and relevant to particular groups of users. For example, the appointments database system in a health care centre is used to enter appointments, view patient details, compile accounts, and send form letters to patients. It can also be used to determine information such as doctors' caseloads, end-of-month receipts, demographics of patients, and so on.

Flat files

At one time, individual departments within hospitals each maintained their own files. Figure 5.1 is a flat file.

Figure 5.1 A flat file

Patient number	First name	Last name	Address	Date of birth
001	Sea	Shore	137 Mast Drive	1/01/1950
002	Tiffany	Light	1839 Leadlight Street	17/07/1976
003	Star	Bright	11 Shining Way	2/05/1968
004	Tuesday	Night	1049 Dark Drive	28/03/1938
005	Pearl	White	16 Treasure Street	22/08/1964
006	Misty	Mountain	13 Steep Road	30/11/1996
007	Will	Fox	33 Forest Road	13/12/1947
008	Spring	Flower	23 Budd Drive	16/10/1990

The amount and complexity of data stored meant that flat files, or single table databases, were usually adequate for most requirements. What this meant, however, was that usually there were multiple files for any individual. A single stay in the hospital might result in files being created in administration, the emergency department, pathology, radiography, and physiotherapy.

Each file would contain the same personal details, together with data specific to the department within which the file was created. This duplication of data used a lot of memory and created problems when files needed to be updated. If a person changed his or her address, for example, it needed to be updated in every file. If any files were missed, then there was a problem with data integrity—there were errors in the data.

The creation of electronic databases using linked tables to organise data was seen as a way to minimises these problems.

Electronic databases

Data stored in a linked table database can be more easily updated, accessed by multiple users and combined in various ways for the purpose of analysis and reporting. It is not the database, however, that performs these functions but the database management system.

Database management system

A database management system (DBMS) is a collection of computer programs designed to store, manage, and retrieve data and information. Microsoft Access is a database management system for small databases, while Oracle is a DBMS for large databases.

There are a number of functions that a DBMS performs to facilitate data management. Table 5.1 outlines these.

Table 5.1 DBMS functions

Function	Description
Storing, retrieving, updating data	The DBMS allows users to store, retrieve, and update data easily and quickly without needing to use complex procedures.
Managing metadata (data dictionary)	The DBMS stores information about the data in the database. This might include type of data stored, meaning of each field in the database, relationship to other data, applications that can access the database, and the functions they can perform.
Data integrity services	The DBMS ensures data integrity by the implementation of pre defined constraints. Examples include limits on the type or length of data that can be entered, restricting the range of values that can be entered, or linking fields. An example would be that a pregnancy test could not be assigned to a male.
Enabling multiple, simultaneous users	The DBMS ensures that errors do not occur as a consequence of two people accessing the same data at the same time.
Backup and recovery services	All systems are subject to failure. In the health care environment, essential services must continue. Therefore it is essential that the DBMS backup and recovery services are able to ensure rapid recovery of the system with minimal impact on the data.
Authorisation and security	Preventing unauthorised access or viewing of unauthorised information. Since health care databases deal with potentially sensitive personal information, this function is vital.

With a DBMS, organisations can control who has access to each part of the system and what operations they can perform. They can create their own data entry forms and screens for different users, tailor queries to report specific data, and adapt the system to meet changing demands relatively easily. A DBMS provides flexibility, security, and ease of use.

Database structures

Structures used for developing multiple, linked tables include hierarchical, network, relational, and object-oriented structures. Each structure is based on the idea of data stored as a set of records. The data structures identify both the data to be stored and the ways in which the data items will be linked to each other.

The earliest linked database structures were hierarchical and network. Both structured data logically and used indexes or pointers to link records. This meant that smaller quantities of data needed to be stored, and records were faster to access. Unfortunately, the process of designing these systems was highly complex and operators needed expert training. Only large and wealthy organisations could afford to use these database systems.

Relational database structures were developed during the 1980s and have become very popular. The relational structure consists of a set of two or more related tables, with a minimum of one shared field between them. The shared field allows the user to shift from one table to another as need be.

This structure of linked tables makes it easier and more efficient to manage large amounts of data and reduces the problems outlined above. Different users are able to view information relevant to them, access to confidential information can be restricted, and data can be easily modified, as it is stored in only one table.

In a relational database, how or where the tables of data are physically stored makes no difference. Each table is identified by a unique name and that name is used by the database to find the table behind the scenes. This is quite different from the hierarchical and network models in which the user requires an understanding of how the data is physically structured within the database in order to retrieve, insert, update, or delete records. The relational structure is therefore easier to understand and use than a hierarchical or network structure. You do not need to be a computer programmer to effectively build and use a relational database. It is probably for this reason that they are very popular systems today.

In recent years, object-oriented databases have become popular. This is partly due to performance difficulties associated with relational databases and partly due to the increased use of databases for storing a greater variety of information such as graphics, sound, video, and images.

Object-oriented databases keep track of objects, which contain both data and action that can be taken on the data. For example, a non-object-oriented general practice database might contain data about patients, such as patient name, address, next scheduled appointment, and, perhaps, medical information such as test results. An object-oriented database would consider patients as objects. All of the data listed above would be associated with each patient, as well as unstructured data such as X-rays. In addition, the object-oriented database would include instructions for processing the data, such as how to calculate and when to print accounts for the various tests.

Although the older hierarchical and network models are considered obsolete, databases built on these models continue to be used in the health care sector today. These older, often very large, databases are referred to as legacy databases. They continue to be used because they often contain data that is integral to the operation of the organisation, and the cost of replacing or redesigning them is prohibitive.

ENABLING DATABASES

Rather than build databases in-house, most organisations, including health care organisations, will contract specialist database designers to do the work in consultation with health professionals and health information managers. One of the first issues for database developers is deciding what to do about existing legacy systems.

Legacy databases

These older systems will have evolved over many years and often perform core functions that cannot be done without a working database. During the life of the database, people will have become familiar with the system. The ntroduction of a new system will require retraining staff. This will be expensive and time consuming, and may be resisted. Productivity may be slowed, at least initially, as staff grapple with the new system and costly errors may be made at this time.

Attempts to transfer from a legacy system to a new database may present incompatibility problems. A new relational or object-oriented database will use very different data structures to a hierarchical or network system. This may require the manual transfer of data from the old to the new system. Given the volume of health care data stored in these legacy databases, this would be an expensive and time-consuming process, with the risk of data being lost or corrupted during the process.

The time, expertise, and expense involved in transferring existing data from a legacy system to a new system tends to see many organisations postponing the decision.

Given the existence of so many legacy systems in the health sector, it would be unusual to find an organisation building a database from scratch. Even where a new database is being developed, it will generally be based on existing data, documents, processes, or procedures. These existing data, documents, and processes will be the basis for analysing the data flows and functions required of the new systems.

Planning

Careful planning will decrease considerably the time involved in constructing and maintaining the database. There are three stages to developing a database:

- *Establishing requirements*: This involves identifying what the users want through the development of an appropriate data model.
- *Designing the database*: During this stage, the data model is translated into tables and relationships. For larger databases, this may involve the development of a data structure diagram.

- *Implementation*: This stage sees the creation of the actual tables and relationships within the database management system.

Establishing requirements

Establishing requirements and building the data model begins with asking questions about:

- *Purpose*: What is the data to be used for?
- *Content*: What data is to be collected?
- *Access*: What data is to be provided to which users?

There will be different views about what the database system should do. From a hospital point of view, a patient-centred health information system is one that is designed around the patient, the data they provide, their needs, and their well-being. From the patient view, a patient-centred system is one that will give them a view of all health information related to them, wherever such information may come from.

It is essential to talk to people who will use the database. A good technique is to brainstorm about the questions they would like the database to answer and the results or reports they would like it to produce. This provides the information to develop a model of user views.

The purpose of a database for a small general practice, for example, may be to maintain individual patient records that incorporate clinical and administrative information, generate accounts, and generate reports and data for government and health insurance requirements. Office staff and general practitioners would, therefore, need to use the database. Each group will have its own specific data requirements:

- *An administrative assistant*: might need the ability to create new patient records, modify existing records, make appointments, and generate accounts.
- *A general practitioner*: may want to view and modify patient records, view summary data for reports, or view financial reports.

These different views of the data are used to create external data models. They identify the data that different groups will need, and which will eventually translate into forms or input screens and reports in the finished database. Therefore, each group of users will have an external data model.

If the purpose of the database has been clearly identified, both the desired outputs (reports, lists, and so on), and the data that needs to be entered into the database to ensure these outputs, will have been identified (client personal information, test results, diagnoses, treatments prescribed) to ensure these outputs.

Designing the database

The different external data models are combined to create a logical data model. The logical model focuses on representing the data as it exists in the 'real world'. Combining information from the various external views allows the database designer to identify the real world items (entities) about which data (attributes) will be collected.

For the general practice database, it can be seen that potential users of the database want information about the *people* who are using medical services. Information must therefore be collected about each person or patient. *Patient* becomes an item, or entity, about which information is stored in the database. For an entity *patient*, users will want to store the name, address, patient number, and so on. These are the attributes of the entity patient, as shown in Figure 5.2.

Figure 5.2 Patient attributes

Medicare no.	First name	Family name	Doctor
0213 4644 2	Fatimah	Khan	Dr Bradley
7834 5711 5	Phat	Nguyen	Dr Grande
3860 9155 3	Julie	Anderson	Dr Grande
7650 5632 7	Anne	Williams	Dr Grande

Another entity in the database might be *doctor*, with the attributes being doctor's identification number, name, room number, and telephone extension, as shown in Figure 5.3.

Figure 5.3 Doctor attributes

ID	Doctor	Room no.	Phone
001	Dr Bradley	25	2256
002	Dr Grande	18	2297

There are a number of guidelines for creating tables in a relational database:

- *Attributes should appear in only one table of the database, with the exception being where an attribute is required to link tables*: Data repeated in more than one table takes up storage space in the computer. This can impact on the speed and efficiency of the database. Duplicate data also means that if any details change, all tables containing that data will need to be amended. This is time consuming and increases the likelihood of errors being made. Each table should only have data that is integral to it.
- *Data must be atomic*: This takes up minimal storage space, allows users to search for information easily and also allows information to be changed in as few fields as possible. Thus, a table will have a field for First Name and Last Name, rather than Name. Address would be in separate fields such as House Number, Street Name, Town, State, and Post Code and so on.
- *Each table in a database needs a 'primary key'*: This enables the database management system to identify the table. Since the primary key needs to be unique, attributes such as names should not generally be used. It is common practice to use codes and ID numbers as primary keys. These are simply added as attributes to each table. In Figure 5.3 the shaded columns are the key attributes. The Medicare

number has been used as the primary key for the *patient* table. This will create problem if, as is sometimes the case, Medicare numbers are allocated to families, rather than to individuals. If this is so, another attribute will need to be identified as the primary key.

Relationships between the various entities can also be identified. Relationships are used to link various tables in the finished database. For example, there will be a relationship, or link, between *patient* and *doctor*, as the patient will see a particular doctor. Therefore, in the finished database, the *patient* table and the *doctor* table will be linked, as shown in Figure 5.4, enabling the user to view the details for the doctor the patient is seeing.

Figure 5.4 Links between relational database tables

Medicare no.	First name	Family name	Doctor
0213 4644 2	Fatimah	Khan	Dr Bradley
7834 5711 5	Phat	Nguyen	Dr Grande
3860 9155 3	Julie	Anderson	Dr Grande
7650 5632 7	Anne	Williams	Dr Grande

Doctor table

Doctor	Room no.	Phone
Dr Bradley	25	2256
Dr Grande	18	2297

For tables to be linked, the same attribute must appear in each. In Figure 5.4, 'Doctor' appears in both tables. The existence of a duplicate attribute creates the relationship between the two entities/tables. The 'Doctor' column in the 'Patient' table is a foreign key. It is an exact match of the primary key in the Doctor table.

There are three possible relationships:

- *One-to-one*: If there is only one doctor in a practice, a one-to-one relationship occurs between Appointment and Patient. An appointment may only have one patient.
- *One-to-many*: The relationship between Patient and Appointment is an example of a one-to-many relationship. There is one patient who may have any number of appointments. This is the preferred relationship in a relational database.
- *Many-to-many*: This relationship indicates that the database is not properly normalised. Where a many-to-many relationship exists, fields should be moved into a new table.

The logical data model enables the database designers to identify:

- *Queries*: The purpose of a database is to store and retrieve information. The query is the primary mechanism for retrieving the information. Queries are questions presented to the database in a predefined format. The results of a query are presented in a new table. In a patient database, for example, you may wish to view all patients who see a particular doctor, have a particular diagnosis, or are members of a particular private medical benefits fund. Queries can access a single table or multiple tables. They are particularly useful when using a relational database because they enable the user to select and combine particular information from multiple tables.
- *Reports*: These are similar to queries in that they retrieve data from one or more tables and display the records. Unlike queries, however, reports allow the inclusion of graphics and the use of backgrounds, different fonts, and other features to create an attractive visual presentation. Reports can be viewed onscreen, or printed.
- *Forms*: Forms are used to make it easier for the user to enter or modify data. Forms clearly identify the fields where each item of data is entered. Forms mean that users do not need to be able to manipulate the underlying structures of the database.

Implementation

The implementation phase involves the creation of the actual tables and relationships within the database management system. If the database is large, this will be undertaken by the database specialist.

MAKING SURE

Usability and security are two important issues for health databases.

Usability

The concept of usability was introduced in Chapter 3. When designing databases, creating user interfaces that make data entry and access easy is a primary usability issue. Issues to consider include:

- *Information density*: This occurs where there is a large amount of information on the screen. Information density can include actual data displayed, but also controls, menu options, text boxes.
- *Lack of location information*: A well-designed database enables the user to easily identify their location. In a patient database, for example, it should be clear exactly which patient the data belongs to.
- *Task interruption*: Prompts or text boxes with reminders or alerts can be useful tools. However, if over-used, these can become irritating and distracting.

- *Changing workflow*: A database may create changes to workflow and routines by requiring data to be entered in a different order to that normally followed.
- *Shifting the burden of work*: Databases, particularly clinical databases for electronic health records, can alter work task responsibility. The reasons and benefits for doing this need to be very clear.

One consequence of a database that is difficult to use is **cognitive overload**. Databases that involve complex steps—those that are performed in an unfamiliar order—or feature high density information displays will require excessive concentration from health professionals. In a hectic work environment where there are already significant demands on the thought processes of the clinician, this may result in cognitive overload. Rosenbaum et al. (1999, p. 1) note:

- Errors in the health environment have the potential to be life threatening to patients.
- The health care profession as a whole has generally been less computer literate than many other industries (although this is now changing).
- The primary focus of health care professionals is on the patient, so computer-based systems receive only secondary attention.

Usability, beginning with database design, requires significant attention.

Security issues for databases

Large relational databases can provide many advantages but there are also some particular difficulties around confidentiality, integrity, and availability of the data. There are technical solutions that, if implemented appropriately, can significantly reduce integrity and availability problems. Confidentiality problems, particularly those around the aggregation of data, are much more difficult to manage as there are few technological solutions that are practical and affordable. This is because it is impossible, at the time a query is made, to work out if the answer to this query, together with other data supplied as a result of previous queries, will provide the missing link that will enable protected data to be inferred. There is some promise that techniques will be developed in future to detect such attacks, but in the meantime the misuse of authorised privileges is a very real threat to maintaining the confidentiality of data.

Availability

There are two availability problems that affect users of databases. One is that their view of the database is unavailable because of system problems. The other is that a particular piece of data is unavailable because it is being used by another user.

A user can be stopped from accessing a particular data item, that they are authorised to access, if this data item is being changed. There would be obvious problems if two community nurses were allowed to book the same car at the same time or an operating theatre was double booked. The mechanism for dealing with this integrity problem involves locking out all other users while a change is being made. It is important to specify the minimum amount of data items that need to be locked and to monitor that the overall system performance is such that most users barely notice that they have been temporarily barred from a piece of data.

Data integrity

Most computer systems these days carefully check the integrity of each piece of data as it is entered into the system. These checks can ensure that data makes sense, but often are not able to check the logical consistency of the whole collection of data.

Although databases have some special problems with integrity maintenance, they also have some special advantages that can help to maintain the integrity of the total collection of data.

Techniques that can be used include:

- use of monitors
- use of constraint rules
- limiting of change actions.

The great advantage of a database can be that it looks after all the data for an entity. This means that some DBMSs allow you to create monitors that trawl through the database looking for inconsistencies in the data. This enables anomalies, such as pregnancy tests on males, to be highlighted and corrected. A monitor, however, will only check for things that it has been told to look for.

Another technique for maintaining the integrity of the data in a database is the use of constraints. These provide overall rules governing how data can exist in a database. Constraints often reflect the structure of an organisation and so need to be rewritten frequently. For example, if you write constraint rules about how many patients of a certain category can be accommodated in a certain ward, and the allowable number changes, you will need to rewrite that constraint rule.

Constraint rules can also be written to check the effect of any changes that can be made to data in a database. For example, if a staff member leaves and you remove him or her from the database, the database can be checked to see if that person is on any mailing lists, has outstanding commitments, is referred to as contact person for any projects and so on.

The final technique that can be used to maintain the integrity of data in a database is to limit the change actions that particular users can perform. A simple divide could be between financial and clinical users: neither group of users should have the ability to alter each other's data. In fact a sophisticated DBMS usually has the ability to discriminate quite finely about what an individual user can read, change, or even know exists.

The main integrity problem that faces databases is when two or more users ask for a piece of data with a view to changing it. Many databases contain data about finite resources: seats on aeroplanes, slots in operating theatres, specialised equipment, or appointment bookings. The problem arises if more than one user asks how many of X at the same time. Each user will have the current value of X returned and at varying intervals of time may or may not choose to use some of X.

Imagine a scenario in which users require prescription pads (X). If X = 4 when Fred, Bill, and Jane enquire at the same time, then there is a problem if both Bill and Jane decide to use one prescription pad each. They may get their prescription pad, but the database may well record three pads left because the change sent by both Bill and Jane was 4 − 1. The simple solution is to allow only one user to see a piece of data at any one time. This is known as data locking. Data locking should be used with care so as not to unnecessarily restrict the ability of users to browse through data.

Because details of medical treatment are considered to be archival records, there is an argument that long-term storage of clinical data prevents the over-writing of records. Various types of 'write once read many' (WORM) drives have been used to retain clinical records since the early 1980s. These WORM drives were originally developed as a type of optical storage; since each type of disc available required its own proprietary reading device, there was no standardisation between WORM systems. More recently, storage on CD-ROM or DVD-ROM has been used for non-erasable storage of data, although there is a likelihood that the integrity of data stored on CD-ROM may diminish after ten years or so.

Box 5.1 illustrates the importance of data integrity.

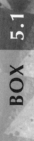

CONSEQUENCE OF INADEQUATE DATA INTEGRITY STANDARDS

BOX 5.1

The death of a young woman from meningitis was thought to be due, at least in part, to her name being spelt in two different ways when it was entered into the hospital computer system. Information was entered in a record created using one spelling. The misspelling of the woman's name at a later time resulted in the creation of a new patient record, and existing information about previous tests and treatments not being identified. As a result, the meningitis was not diagnosed and the young woman was not treated (Fleet 1998).

Data confidentiality

The principal aim for data confidentiality in a health care system is to avoid disclosing information that can cause people harm while at the same time enabling disclosure of information for the primary purpose for which data is usually supplied: to manage the health care or the employment of the individuals that the data describes. The challenge lies not so much in protecting the direct disclosure of personally identified data to unauthorised users, but in protecting against users being able to work out some or all of this data from responses to legitimate queries. This partial disclosure can be in the following forms:

- a non-negative result to a 'how many' query, for example tests for a certain disease or class of diseases
- the name of an unexpected field in a table, for example sick days off without a certificate
- the result of carefully crafted inference attacks.

As Box 5.2 illustrates, ensuring confidentiality of medical information is extremely important.

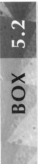

THE IMPORTANCE OF CONFIDENTIALITY

On 6 June 2004, the *Sydney Morning Herald* reported the case of a patient whose medical records had been published on the Internet as a result of hospital error. The records contained highly sensitive information, including psychiatric details and treatment related to her sexuality. The paper reported that other patient files were also published on the Internet, some of which contained details regarding HIV status (Teutsch 2004).

Inference attacks

Imagine a hospital database that protected the name, address, and contact details of individual staff to all but approved applications and a few users. However, many users could obtain addresses and telephone numbers so long as they could not be tied to an individual. The challenge is for a patient to find out the address of a particular male nurse. First the patient has to find out how to authenticate to the system. Perhaps a post-it note will be stuck next to the terminal, maybe some shoulder surfing will help, or maybe guessing 'Ward X' and password 'staff' will do? Access to the database achieved, a direct request for the address of person x should be refused. Similarly a request for the address of male nurses in Ward X might be refused, as there may be only one data item contributing to the reply. However, two queries for the addresses of 'nurses in Ward E' and 'female nurses in Ward X' would allow you to extract the address of the male nurse in Ward X quite easily. If there were several male nurses in Ward X, then queries that differentiated groups of nurses by shift or age could help reduce the possibilities to only one.

This is a simple example of what can be sophisticated attacks worked out with the help of logic and set algebra. The attacker has the time to make these calculations, but there is no way that the database software can do the same in order to detect that a series of legitimate queries could be breaking confidentiality. This is especially true if the attacker submits the queries over an extended period of time. Unfortunately, defences such as only providing counts, sums, ranges, and averages for numerical data can be circumvented in a similar way.

The defences against these attacks are not very useful if data accuracy is required. They involve changing the data such that it is fit for the purpose required but changed in some way. For example, address information may be changed to only the name of the nearest main road, bus stop, or postcode. This needs special care in health applications as usually data needs to be precise. However, the need for precision declines with the age of the data, and altering or *sanitising* older data may be useful.

This can be a particularly useful defence against some *aggregation* attacks. These try to retrieve all the available data about an individual in order to work out the wanted information. However, being able to retrieve such data is precisely one of the benefits a centralised system can deliver to clinicians faced with a difficult diagnosis. In this case sanitised data would defeat a legitimate purpose.

The particular vulnerabilities in relational databases, especially those that allow a leaking of confidential medical data, highlight the importance of good authentication practices and other security measures such as physical access control.

SUMMARY

Databases are a fundamental tool for health information management. They have applications in clinical, research, education, and management areas. Databases may function as repositories of information, such as Medline, or they may function as information management tools.

Databases have evolved from flat files through hierarchical, network, relational, and object-oriented structures. Relational database structures are common today, although many health care organisations still use legacy systems based on hierarchical and network structures.

Electronic databases utilise database management systems, which are a collection of programs designed to store, manage, and retrieve data and information. Database management systems also include programs to manage multiple access, data integrity and authorisation, and security functions.

Planning and implementing a database should be a consultative process involving not only database specialists but also end-users. The first phase involves identifying user output needs. Different groups of users will have different output needs. Therefore, there will be several user views, or external data models. External data models form the basis of the forms, queries, and reports that the database will use.

External data models are combined to form the logical data model. The logical data model focuses on representing data as it exists in the real world. This enables the database designer to identify the tables (entities) and attributes required. There will be more than one table in a relational database. Each will contain information about a specific entity. Tables are linked using primary keys. Each table has a primary key. The primary key is an attribute that must be unique for each entity. For this reason names do not make good primary keys.

The logical data model is used to build the physical database. This is usually the responsibility of the database specialist.

To ensure the database is effective, attention needs to be paid to usability aspects including establishing parameters for data types to facilitate ease of data entry, and design aspects of the user interface. Security must also be considered. In a database, security issues focus on availability, data integrity, and confidentiality.

WWW LINKS

Geekgirl's plain English computing: database tutorial <http://www.geekgirls.com/>
Health InfoDesign <http://www.healthinfodesign.com/>

CRITICAL THINKING

The community nurses and allied health professionals working out of the Global Village Community Health Centre are seeking to improve information sharing as they work together to support older residents with chronic health problems. Currently, the community nurses and each allied health area maintain their own records, and information is shared at case conferences. Much of this information could be more efficiently communicated using a database management system, which would allow health professionals to merge and share their data and information. The database would be located on the Centre server, and each professional would access the data from their own workstation.

1 Who might be the main user groups for this database?
2 What might be the data requirements for each user group? Consider data to be collected and data to be presented to the user.
3 Design some screens for data entry and information reports, applying usability guidelines.
4 What technical and human security safeguards might be required for the database?

CHAPTER 6

HEALTH INFORMATION SYSTEMS

OVERVIEW

While there is a perception in some circles today that health informatics is about the management of clinical data and information, in reality, the discipline deals with the management of all health data and information. The earliest applications of information systems in most health services were primarily for administration. As a result, in many health services today you will find that administrative information/knowledge management systems tend to be more widely used, more sophisticated and more readily accepted than clinical applications.

This chapter focuses on the administrative systems. Clinical systems are discussed in later chapters.

OBJECTIVES

At the completion of this chapter, you should be able to:
- describe applications of information systems in the health care environment
- discuss factors shaping the development of health information systems
- discuss models used in information systems planning
- outline life cycle models
- list critical success factors and outline their importance for successful development of information systems
- discuss standards relevant to health information systems.

CONCEPTS

Information system
Health information system

INTRODUCTION

Although technology is widely assumed to be an integral component of information systems, this is not necessarily the case. From a systems-theory perspective, information systems are interrelated components of people, data, and work procedures interacting in established patterns to collect, process, manage, and communicate health data and information to achieve specific goals. This may include procedures and processes that are manual, computer based, or a combination of both. Information systems existed long before the advent of information and communications technologies. Therefore, while information systems today are increasingly automated, many organisations continue to rely on paper-based manual or partially automated systems.

Excellent, you say. Here is a golden opportunity for the health informatics professional to automate, integrate, and bring these organisations into the twenty-first century. Maybe so, but this will require an understanding of the factors contributing to successful implementation of information systems. This includes understanding the scope and levels of decision-making facilitated by information systems, the planning processes, tools, and techniques used in information systems development and the technical, cultural, and organisational factors shaping their development and operation.

This chapter explores these areas. It begins by discussing the way information systems are used in the health care environment. The processes, tools, and techniques used to develop health information systems are discussed, including an analysis of cultural, organisational, and technical issues. Finally, issues around managing the development and use of health information systems are considered.

USING HEALTH INFORMATION SYSTEMS

> The delivery of health care is built on information systems (Johns 2002, p. 22).

Health information systems have been developing since medical care began to be institutionalised in the nineteenth century. Electronic systems have been slowly making inroads into the health environment since the 1960s. From the 1970s to the mid-1990s, they were used internally by organisations, initially within departments but increasingly across departments to an enterprise level. A logical extension from this inward focus, and a response to an increasing emphasis on coordinated and integrated health care, has seen organisations turn outwards to explore the potential for information sharing with each other. Today, information systems are used to support information management and decision-making activities in policy and planning, patient care, education, and research within and across organisations. Systems are many and varied and a number of classification systems are used to convey this complexity.

What are we talking about?

An information system

An information system consists of data, people, technology, procedures, and communication channels that interact to gather, record, process, store, and report information within and between organisations. Examples of information systems run the gamut from simple and informal devices (pencil and paper or hardware) and communication channels (word of mouth) to complex hardware devices (super-computers) and formal communication channels (the Internet and intranets). The latter computer-based information systems (CBIS) are the focus of this chapter.

Figure 6.1 depicts the components of a computer-based information system.

Figure 6.1 Components of a computer-based information system

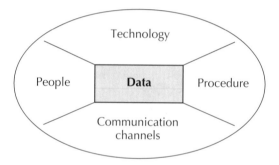

The components are:

- *People*: business personnel (sponsors who request the systems and end-users who capture, input, report, and use the data) and information systems (IS) personnel (who analyse and develop the systems)
- *Technology*: physical devices (hardware) that facilitate the interaction of the other components
- *Procedures*: the instructions (software) needed to perform the various functions for which the system is intended (in an automated information system, the technology would be the hardware and the procedures would be explicated by the software or computer programs)
- *Communication channels*: the networks or mechanisms through which the information is moved from one physical device to another
- *Data*: the raw facts and figures that are central to the purpose of the system.

These five components work together to effect three simple actions—input, process, output—to transform raw data into useful information that can be used to make management decisions. Business and IS personnel must work together to determine the nature of each of the five components and the way in which they interact.

Health information systems

In the health care environment, information systems may be differentiated in terms of their clinical, administrative, education, research, and other health-related functions. This is a rather simplistic classification, however, since there is considerable overlap and blurring of functions. Beaumont (1999, p. 5), for example, notes that 'it is basically impossible to develop any clinical system without it depending on some type of administrative data'.

Information systems may also be differentiated according to their purpose. This gives:

- *Transaction processing systems (TPS)*: (payroll, inventory, admission, and discharge), and office automation systems (word processors, spreadsheets, email systems for daily activities, and communication)
- *Management information systems (MIS)*: provide information to enable managers to perform their daily work
- *Decision support systems (DSS)*: provide information, models, and data-manipulation tools to assist with decision-making
- *Expert systems (ES)*: support decision-making by organising facts and knowledge into rules that are applied to a given set of questions or symptoms.

Classifying systems in this way gives an indication of the spread of information systems across the health care environment. Information systems are also employed at different levels within the organisation from strategic through tactical to operational decision-making. Strategic decision-making identifies the broad goals and functions of the organisation. Tactical decision-making establishes how these goals will be achieved, while operational decision-making plans the day-to-day activities needed to achieve the goals. To support this process, strategic information systems draw on the output from tactical information systems, which, in turn, draw on operational systems.

Figure 6.2 combines these various classifications of health information systems into a matrix.

The matrix gives a clearer picture of the depth and breadth of health information systems across the health care environment. For example:

- *Financial information systems*: range from transaction-processing functions undertaken by specific individuals or work groups to financial decision support systems for strategic decisions around investment management, capital budgeting, and financial planning.
- *Clinical information systems*: include sophisticated organisation-wide systems and systems suited to specific environments such as acute care, or to specific disciplines such as surgery or obstetrics.
- *Nursing information systems*: include systems used to develop patient care plans, to expert systems and decision support systems.

Figure 6.2 Levels and types of information systems

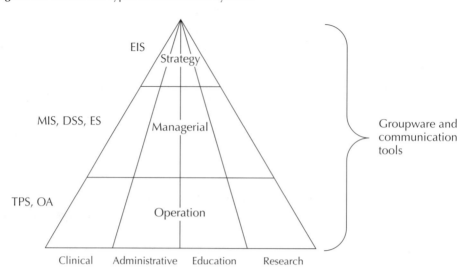

Applications of information systems

Early uses of electronic systems in health were driven by financial considerations, and the methods used were developed from hospital accounting and billing systems. In 1994, Tan and Hanna found that the use of IT in health care was primarily focused on transaction processing and management control in areas of administration such as accounting, payroll, and inventory.

The most vigorous developments were in the USA, where commercial influences in the health system were the strongest. Most hospital visits were billable, and it was essential to make sure that all chargeable components of the episode were recorded correctly, and invoiced to the appropriate payer. In the United Kingdom, and to a lesser extent in Australia, hospital activity was funded centrally, and there was much less impetus to collect detailed data about elements of hospital care to populate billing systems. Most hospital systems were designed to automate one or two functions, and the data structures used were set up with little consideration given to possible expansion into other areas of hospital activity. As modules were expanded and additional modules written, the underlying logic of the overall application became more and more convoluted. Documentation of code often lagged behind development, and made the applications difficult to support and maintain.

Over the decades, health information systems have evolved to enable increasing functionality and integration, yet the use of these systems varies widely from one health enterprise to another. Many small enterprises are still coming to grips with operational information systems, while large national systems such as Health Canada are well advanced in the development of strategic information systems. Most organisations use a combination of systems, still using paper for some processes, and having a mix of old and new electronic systems. Box 6.1 describes the implementation of an information system that continues to use paper processes.

BOX 6.1

IMPLEMENTATION OF AN INFORMATION SYSTEM

Honolulu based Straub Clinic and Hospital, part of Hawaii Pacific Health, included a 159-bed hospital, 14 neighbourhood clinics, 200 physicians, and 32 specialists. The challenge was to move patient charts, information, and administrative data between different islands. Existing medical data management, and workflow systems relied on paper-based charts, which limited the ability to track clinical information. Workflow included dictated notes, which were distributed, reviewed, and signed; lab and radiology reports, which were distributed, reviewed, and initialled; and letters intended for referring physicians.

Straub wanted to improve the entire system of workflow but did not want to move to a full electronic health record. After some consideration, the hospital adopted a web-based, open solution for clinical messaging from Axolotl Corp. Mountain View, California. Called Elysium, this system automatically delivers results from the existing system to physicians' desktop computers. They are then able to annotate and store information in patient charts, either in electronic or paper form. Physicians and nurses receive electronic transcriptions, and lab and radiology reports. Physicians review dictation on their PC, and edit and electronically sign and deliver these to the health information department for printing and filing into medical records. Lab results are displayed in email format and are available for review as soon as they are complete, and abnormal results are flagged for immediate attention. The system has seen a reduction in administrative time and costs related to tracking lost and delayed results, and a reduction in document-management costs. The facility is now planning to pilot mobile systems, also from Axolotl Corp. These mobile systems will enable physicians to review lab reports and manage clinical information, view cumulative information, write prescriptions and communicate with their staff from a handheld computer.

Adapted from Glenn & Chung, Health Management Technology, January 2003
(http://www.healthmgttech.com/)

ENABLING HEALTH INFORMATION SYSTEMS

Enormous investment has gone into computerised hospital information systems worldwide. Yet the overall benefits and costs of hospital information systems have rarely been assessed (Littlejohns et al. 2003, p. 860).

It is accepted that there have been many more health information system failures than successes. One of two major reasons for cancelling an information systems project is poor planning and management (Engelbardt & Nelson 2002, p. 162). Planning ensures that the system is consistent with the overall strategic goals of the organisation and ensures a systematic approach to implementation and evaluation.

Strategic planning for information systems

> In order for any organisation to be successful, its information resources must support critical functions and strategic objectives. Thus the planning for information systems must be based on the knowledge of the health-care organisations and its critical goals or success factors (Johns 2002, p. 101).

Perhaps as a legacy from its project-based past, or perhaps in response to the professional and departmental silos characteristic of the health environment, health information systems development has tended to adopt an 'episodic' approach, focusing on the immediate system requirements with little attention paid to wider organisational or health system trends and requirements. Recent trends towards strategic planning for information systems are broadening this focus, encouraging developers of individual systems to view them as part of a larger potentially integrated environment.

Strategic planning for IT systems is challenging enough, but developing IT strategies for health care organisations is particularly complex and has a higher chance of being rejected than is the case in commercial organisations. There are two reasons for this. The first is the complex structures with different lines of responsibility and management, which are characteristic of health care. The second is the goal of improving the delivery of health care, which is additional to the usual focus on cost justifications present in commercial organisations.

As an enterprise-wide approach, strategic planning facilitates the development of integrated information systems by identifying the information needs of the organisation as a whole. Although the reality for many health organisations may still be somewhat less than enterprise-wide systems, planning still needs to be considered in the context of the strategic goals and overall direction. Individual systems can then be planned and implemented with a view to their eventual integration into an enterprise-wide system. A crucial step in this process is the analysis of the environment into which the system will be introduced.

The health care environment

> The term *health care* is a deceptively simple one embracing multiple, inherently complex sets of processes and interactions. This complexity strongly influences the application of health care information systems (Norris 2002, p. 205).

Characteristics of the health care environment that impact on the development of a system include:

- specialisation and departmentalisation
- the nature of health data and information

- work processes
- technologies: the legacy of the technological past.

Specialisation and departmentalisation

We just cannot get away from the cultural and organisational characteristics of the health care environment. We have seen how the increasing complexity of medical and health knowledge resulted in specialisation and departmentalisation of the health care system. This influenced the development of information systems, which initially focused on isolated areas and problems. Systems were created to serve a particular purpose within specific departments. A plethora of data systems, databases, software, and reporting mechanisms were developed. The majority of these were developed or purchased independently of one another and were often unable to communicate with other programs or applications. As a result, information systems became information silos, locking data within one system, department, or organisation and making it unavailable to other parts of the organisation or service.

The nature of health data and information

Health information is multi-faceted, complex, and widely distributed. It ranges from individual patient information, collected and stored by a single health professional, to aggregate information, combining many sets of individual details and stored in large health databases. It can include clinical information, such as test results, and administrative information, such as health insurance numbers. It can reside in a wide range of locations, including health care organisations, government departments and agencies, educational and research institutions, and non-government and private organisations. Use of health information can range from the macro level, where aggregate data is used for policy, strategic planning, research, and education, to the micro level, where individual patient information is used for decisions regarding treatment and services. These characteristics mean that data and information in health information systems are very different to that in the business and commercial environment. Table 6.1 highlights these differences.

The nature of health and medical information creates particular problems for integrated information systems. Since the object of developing increasingly integrated systems is to facilitate information sharing, we need to overcome the problem of incompatible data. The development of standards is intended to do this. Standards currently being developed in health informatics were discussed in Chapter 4. They are discussed in greater detail in the section 'Controlling IT' later in this chapter.

Work processes

The introduction of an information system into a health environment can impact on both personal routines and the more formal routines utilised by many within the enterprise. As enterprise systems incorporate more and more clinical routines, this is likely to become an increasingly critical element to be considered. Examples include:

Table 6.1 Differences in financial system data and health care system data

Financial system	Health care system
Information is well structured.	While administrative information may be clearly structured, health and medical information is complex and difficult to structure.
The number of possible transactions is limited.	A large number of different transactions possible.
Vocabularies and terminology is limited.	Vocabularies and terminologies are many and varied.
Well-established standards exist for data exchange between institutions.	Standards may exist for financial and administrative data exchange. However, for other health and medical information, much work remains to be done.
Records contain few, simple data types.	Data types are disparate and complex.
Transactions are easy—customers can perform many themselves.	Transactions need to be completed by a professional.

Source: adapted from Altman 1997.

- Some routines for pulling patient files, adding new data, and replacing the file will move from the physical environment to the virtual environment. This may result in different individuals being responsible for the steps, or having to use different methods for completing their tasks.
- In an environment such as a hospital, where the clinician enters information on charts located in proximity to the patient, an electronic record system may require the use of a data entry devices not so conveniently located or easy to use.

While electronic systems may have advantages, existing routines will have evolved to suit the particular working environment or the particular preferences of each health professional. Generally, those who follow the routines feel comfortable doing so. It is therefore understandable that there may be resistance to the changes, particularly if the advantages are not immediately clear.

There may also be conflicting views about the advantages of a new system. From an administrative perspective, for example, a change in the person who collects data may be viewed as an increase in efficiency, yet the health professional who is required to collect additional information may view the proposed system as impacting on quality of service.

Technologies: the legacy of the technological past

Health organisations began to use information technology during the 1960s, primarily to automate existing paper-based financial and administrative processes and procedures. As the technology developed, these automated processes evolved into more complex information systems. Requirements or opportunities for increased communication between departments saw many systems re-jigged or customised. Many of these solutions were short term, ad hoc, and expensive.

Today, the existing IT infrastructure in many organisations is a web of interconnected information silos often running on obsolete hardware and outdated software. They are time consuming and expensive to maintain, with a lack of documentation and few, if any, technical staff with any knowledge of how their system is structured and operates. Yet, while they may be cumbersome, slow, and perhaps subject to downtime, these systems represent considerable financial investment, are already installed, people know how to work them, and they often perform essential operations that cannot be done without a working computer system. Although increasingly unable to meet current information-sharing requirements, they influence, even limit, choices relating to new systems and processes. Nevertheless, for the last decade there has been increasing interest in the development of health information systems that span the enterprise and beyond. 'Today's vision must be toward fully integrated systems supported by flexible data models, communication technologies, and tools that enhance decision-making, improve quality and productivity, and reduce administrative costs' (Johns 2002, p. 86). Yet, while this may be the vision, the reality for many organisations is the need to adapt, develop, or integrate existing older systems in a changing environment. So begins the planning process.

Planning

> The track record for strong planning within IT environments has not been overwhelming. More than 10 per cent of all IT projects are undertaken with no formal planning (Engelbardt & Nelson 2002, p. 162).

Although there are many health and hospital information systems available on the market today, very few are able to meet all the requirements of an organisation or department or offer the level of integration increasingly expected by health systems. It is therefore standard practice to buy software, which is then designed, built, and customised for the specific organisation. Whether building or buying, it is widely accepted that successful development and implementation of an information system requires careful planning.

Prior to the 1960s, systems developers relied on experience and rule-of-thumb. The emphasis at this time was on computerising manual systems, which would simply mirror and support the existing paper-based information system. Programming was considered essential, while systems analysis was not. Unfortunately, this often meant that the needs of the users were not clearly identified and the information system was sometimes not appropriate for its purpose. In response to these problems, formal life-cycle approaches and structured methods in information systems design and development began to be used. While the systems development lifecycle (SDLC) is still considered to have some advantages, particularly for larger projects, it is often found to be too inflexible, too slow, or too ineffective in today's health care environment. We are therefore seeing the increasing use of alternative methodologies such as **rapid applications development (RAD)**. One way of exploring the differences between these approaches is by using Eric Raymond's analogy of the cathedral and the bazaar. This is summarised in Box 6.2. Table 6.2 summarises the differences between the two approaches.

Of the health information system projects in development today, most can readily be categorised as either cathedral or bazaar developments. Cathedral projects often have a scope that seems to have ignored the intended end-users in the early phases of development. The pace of development often appears ponderous.

BOX 6.2 THE CATHEDRAL AND THE BAZAAR

Eric Raymond wrote about the differences between conventional application development, and the norms that apply to developments that take place in the open source community. He writes about his own experiences developing a fetchmail mail transport utility, but his observations have relevance to the approach taken by many health departments and organisations to the development of health information systems.

The title of the paper, 'The Cathedral and the Bazaar', captures the essential differences between the two approaches. 'The most important software...needed to be built like cathedrals, carefully crafted by individual wizards or small bands of mages working in splendid isolation, with no beta to be released before its time' (Raymond 2000, p. 1). A cathedral is commissioned by a small powerful group, who may not have a lot in common with those who will use it. It is designed by experts who are expected to know all about designing and building edifices. Artisans create the product over a long period, and are protective of their work, unwilling to expose it to review until they are happy with their work. 'Linus Torvalds's style of development—release early and often, delegate everything you can, be open to the point of promiscuity—came as a surprise. No quiet, reverent cathedral-building here—rather...a great babbling bazaar of differing agendas and approaches...out of which a coherent and stable system could seemingly emerge only by a succession of miracles' (Raymond 2000, p. 2). A bazaar product is developed close to its intended users. They watch the process, try early versions of the product, and comment and perhaps contribute to the work.

Table 6.2 Differences between cathedral and bazaar

Feature	Cathedral	Bazaar
Cost	High	Moderate to low
Development time	Long (sometimes years)	Short (months)
Risk of failure	Low to moderate	Moderate to high
Impact of failure	Considerable	Small
Embarrassment caused by failure	Considerable	Little or none
Specification and design	Fixed, linear, detailed; prepared in advance	May be sketchy; iterative —develops as work progresses
Ownership	High level	Low level (close to users)
Flexibility	Low	High
Control	Tight, central	Relaxed, near end-users

The cathedral: the HIS development life cycle

Since the early 1970s, information systems developers have utilised a methodology variously referred to as conventional systems analysis, the systems development life cycle (SDLC), or the waterfall model. Although this model is now considered by many to have passed its 'use-by' date, it nevertheless provides a useful indication of the range of activities and processes involved in the development of an information system. Therefore we will briefly outline the traditional information systems methodology, discuss criticisms of the 'pure' model, and introduce some modified approaches that have been used in the design and development of health information systems.

The systems development life cycle consists of several phases. These are the same whether the system is being built in-house, or purchased as an off-the-shelf program and modified. The difference is that coding and debugging are replaced by evaluation of the potential of purchased products, and purchase of the software. Table 6.3 summarises the systems development life cycle.

The bazaar: rapid applications development (RAD)

Rapid applications development (RAD) is an approach to systems development that is designed to provide fast development with better quality results than the traditional waterfall approach. The main elements of RAD are:

- *User involvement*: Every RAD team includes at least one full-time user participant.
- *Rapid design*: The methodology requires that a fully functioning system be delivered in 60 to 120 days. This limits both the size and type of projects that can be carried out successfully with RAD. The development of complex technical systems is

Table 6.3 Systems development life cycle

Phase	Purpose
Feasibility study	A preliminary investigation that seeks to determine whether the organisation has a problem and whether that problem can be solved by an information system.
System design	Focuses on how to implement the requirements identified in the previous phase and will describe in detail the desired features and operations of the system. This will include screen layouts, business rules, process diagrams, and other documentation.
System construction	Building of the system. It includes setting up the databases and networks, coding and testing programs, establishing or installing new hardware and software, writing the documentation, and testing the system.
Implementation	The final steps needed to make the new or modified system operational, including conversion of data from the old to the new system, final testing, and training users.
Review and maintenance	Using and evaluating the system after it has been installed and is in use.

difficult, if not impossible, with such a time frame, unless larger systems can be divided into sections and developed separately.

- *Prototyping*: The development team produces a working prototype of the system, usually in a matter of days. Each prototype is tested by users, and returned to the development team for reworking, at which point the cycle repeats.
- *Iteration*: Prototypes are reviewed and modified and then reviewed again. This enables the rapid evolution of a final version fully acceptable to users.
- *Time limits*: The entire project is controlled by prioritising development elements and defining delivery deadlines. If projects start to lag behind the time lines, the emphasis is on reducing the requirements, not increasing the deadlines.
- *Rapid development tools*: RAD relies on the use of tools such as fourth generation languages (4GL), graphical user interface (GUI) builders, database management systems (DBMS), and computer-aided software engineering (CASE) tools.
- *Practical acceptability as a key measure of success*: The completed system needs to be acceptable to end-users.

RAD was initially used to build smaller information systems, and was considered more appropriate for these than for larger, complex systems of the type beginning to emerge in the health sector. However, the approach has also been successfully applied to larger administrative systems. The large system is broken into separate parts and the parts of the system are developed, tested, and adjusted one at a time.

The method is still considered unsuitable for unique and/or highly complex programs, which must be hand-designed and coded. Table 6.4 summarises RAD phases.

Table 6.4 Phases of rapid applications development

Requirements planning	Defines the information system requirements, obtains sponsor approval and commitment, and plans the further implementation of the project.
User design	Uses the requirements documents to design the system architecture, software components, interfaces, and databases. Health professionals who will use the system participate in this phase.
Construction	Developing, testing, and revising the system. The design is implemented using the iterative prototype cycle, enabling end-users to review and comment as the system is developed.
Cutover	Sees the system installed. It involves a number of different activities including installation of the new system and conversion of the old system, comprehensive testing, training of end-users, and dealing with organisational changes arising from the new system. This may involve changes to workflows and routines and also to roles and responsibilities.

Planning tools: modelling

In Chapter 5, modelling was discussed in the context of database design. Modelling is also valuable tool for information systems development. Modelling can be used for:

- *Data*: in the development of a logical database design. The data model provides a graphical picture of the organisation's data needs, enabling the development of the information systems master plan.
- *Processes*: by identifying and depicting the activities or processes of the organisation.

At the enterprise level, the data model 'considers the goals of the enterprise, identifies data requirements, identifies activities or processes to be supported, and sets priorities for implementation' (Johns 2002, p. 162). At the system level, the data model describes the purpose of the application and provides detailed descriptions of the data required.

Data modelling

The purpose of data modelling is to produce a description, usually in diagrammatic form, of the data and information needed to support the activities of the organisation. It is a map showing what data is being used (or will be used), where it will be kept and how it is related. Data models should raise and answer questions such as:

- What are the categories of data?
- Who needs access?
- Who should serve as stewards?
- Where should data reside and flow?

There are three categories of data model:

- *The conceptual data model*: focuses on representing the data as the user sees it in the 'real world' and therefore requires end-user input. It is essentially a mental model that describes all relevant information that is currently available, or that will be used by the organisation in the future, about entities of interest (person, place, or thing—for example, patient, invoice, department). It also shows the relationships that exist between the entities. The conceptual model can also be referred to as an entity–relationship (E–R) diagram. Figure 6.3 is a simple conceptual model (where a patient has one address and an address can be attributed to many patients).

Figure 6.3 Simple conceptual data model

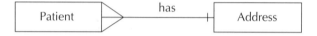

- *The logical data model*: looks at the data within the system from the perspective of specific groups of users and represents data in a format that is meaningful to the user and to the software programs that process the data. In every system, there are several groups of users, each with their own specific data flows and requirements and, therefore, with their own particular perspective on the conceptual model. There can be an endless number of logical models—one specifically tailored to every individual user or group of users. All logical models are derived from the conceptual data model. Clearly the logical data model requires considerable input from end-users, allowing the users to see database information in a non-technical way. Figure 6.4 shows a logical data model.

Figure 6.4 Simple logical data model

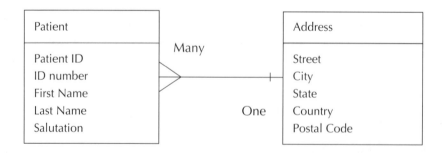

- *The physical data model*: is concerned with the structure of the data and how it is physically arranged and organised in the databases. It is used by database developers to make efficient use of storage, manipulation, and retrieval mechanisms. It illustrates the technical aspects of the system and usually does not involve end-users or health informatics professionals (unless they have expertise in systems design and/or database design). Figure 6.5 shows a simple physical data model.

Figure 6.5 Simple physical data model

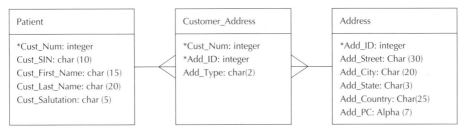

Patient	Customer_Address	Address
*Cust_Num: integer Cust_SIN: char (10) Cust_First_Name: char (15) Cust_Last_Name: char (20) Cust_Salutation: char (5)	*Cust_Num: integer *Add_ID: integer Add_Type: char(2)	*Add_ID: integer Add_Street: Char (30) Add_City: Char (20) Add_State: Char(3) Add_Country: Char(25) Add_PC: Alpha (7)

Process modelling

While the data model identifies data that will exist in the systems databases, it does not indicate the processes the system will perform on the data. Process modelling provides this information.

The main tool of process modelling is the data flow diagram. This shows the flow of data through a system and the processing performed on the data by that system. Figure 6.6 is a simplified data flow model for a general practice.

Figure 6.6 Simple data flow model

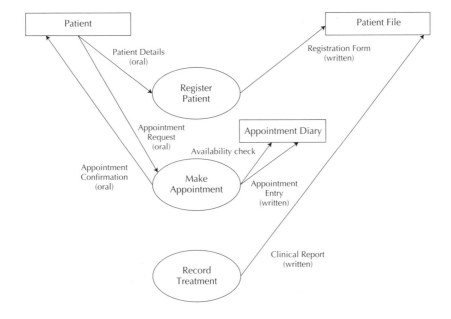

This data flow diagram (DFD) shows three processes. In reality there would be many more processes, including producing accounts, receiving payments, making referrals, and so on. Diagrams would be drawn to show each process in detail. A computer science or systems analysis textbook or website will provide detailed information about data flow diagrams.

Object-oriented modelling

> Developers...realised that systems could be more efficiently developed if both process and data were handled simultaneously (Johns 2002, p. 188).

It is very difficult to balance both data and process models. This is particularly true of complex information systems and higher level planning. Object-oriented modelling is an approach that incorporates both data and process modelling.

Some key elements of object-oriented modelling include:

- *Objects*: An object is a person, place, event, or item. Each object has specific attributes and behaviours. For example, each object patient can change addresses or appointment times.
- *Classes*: Objects are grouped into classes that share a common structure, and common behaviour. Classes therefore distinguish one type of object from another. In a hospital information system, each individual patient (object) belongs to the class patient.
- *Inheritance*: Objects and classes are arranged hierarchically.

Critical success factors (CSFs)

> When systems are evaluated, about three-quarters are considered to have failed, and there is no evidence that they improve the productivity of health professionals (Littlejohns et al. 2003, p. 860).

In any organisation, department, or industry, there will be certain critical factors that, if achieved, will result in success, but if not achieved, the organisation, department, or industry will experience serious difficulties. These are known as critical success factors (CSFs). They are the few key areas where things must go right if the overall project is to be successful, and should therefore receive constant and careful attention.

Just as there are various levels of strategic planning—organisation, department, project—so too are there various levels of critical success factor analysis with higher levels informing lower levels. For health information systems, strategic critical success factors should provide the guiding direction for the development of systems and applications and the use of information technology. This is shown in Table 6.5.

Although critical success factors vary from project to project, research suggests that there are a number of CSFs that are relevant to most projects. These include:

- a federal approach
- senior management support
- project champion
- project management
- project team membership
- end-user input and participation
- change management
- communication
- end-user skill development.

Table 6.5 Hierarchy of critical success factors

Level	Goal	CSFs
Organisation strategic plan	Improve positive patient outcomes by 10 per cent	More accurate diagnosis Improve education
IS department strategic plan	Develop system to improve patient outcomes	Links to external data Links to internal data Provide modelling, expert systems, and decision support capabilities
Project	Provide modelling, expert systems, and decision support capabilities	Top management support Project management User involvement

A federal approach

> One of the main factors associated with enterprise systems failure is lack of integration (Sumner 1999, p. 299).

A federal approach involves the identification of information requirements for the organisation as a whole before the specific needs of particular departments or groups of health professionals are considered. The process begins at the strategic planning level. This ensures that information systems are aligned with the organisation's overall strategic directions and that department- or function-specific systems will be able to be integrated as enterprise-wide systems emerge.

Senior management support

Executive level support is a critical success factor since senior management support will confirm that the project is consistent with strategic goals. Senior management support should also ensure that the required resources are available and may facilitate acceptance at lower levels within the organisation. Where the project is an enterprise system that impacts on different groups and departments, and cuts across traditional boundaries, roles, and authority, senior management may be required to negotiate or arbitrate between the affected parties.

Project champion

The importance of a project champion has long been acknowledged as a success factor for many types of innovation and change within an organisation. A project champion is considered critical for successful information systems development. A project champion, who is in a position to (formally or informally) influence opinion, will be instrumental in developing acceptance. A project champion at senior management level will be particularly conducive to success.

Project management

> A botched project is one of the major reasons users get turned off to technology (Overby 2002, p. 1).

Project management is responsible for the planning, development and implementation of a project. When it is considered that one of two major reasons for cancelling an information systems project is poor planning and management, it becomes clear that good management will be a critical success factor. Project management includes both the people and the processes (Engelbardt & Nelson 2002, p. 162). As an enterprise-wide project will cut across departments and professional areas of responsibility, the project manager will need to have sufficient authority to enable him or her to work across departmental or inter-professional boundaries. Strong project management skills including the ability to select an appropriate planning methodology and to manage the project in a systematic and controlled manner are also attributes of a good manager.

Project team membership

The project team will have the responsibility for developing and implementing the system and interacting with and training end-users. Therefore, the membership of the team will be a critical element in the success of the project. Several characteristics have been identified as contributing to a successful project team. Project team members need to be drawn from both the IT/IS area and the various departments and professional groups who will be using the system. All team members do not need to work full-time on the project. Given the nature of health care, this would be almost impossible. However, there does need to be a core team dedicated full-time to the project. It may be difficult to find staff willing to commit full-time. Where incentives or rewards for participation are offered, recruitment is often more successful. This underlines the critical nature of top management support.

End-user input/participation

End-user involvement helps to ensure that the system will meet end-user needs. End-user involvement may also facilitate acceptance of any changes to work routines and work habits. The use of rapid applications development provides the opportunity for greater end-user involvement. For more traditional life cycle methods, advisory groups and committees facilitate end-user participation.

Change management

> They may not be afraid of technology. They may not even be afraid of change. But they're afraid of poorly managed change (Overby 2002, p. 1).

The introduction of an electronic information system will generally involve significant change. Therefore, an effective change management strategy should be part of project planning. Change management strategies should begin early in the project and continue throughout the entire life cycle. The change management strategy should also match the organisation culture (see Chapter 3).

Communication

Extensive user involvement will ensure effective communication. Where user participation is limited, people should be kept informed at every stage of the project. Input and feedback should also be sought from users. Good communication will help to ensure that expectations about the system are realistic and accurate.

End-user skill development

User acceptance will be enhanced if users experience success using the new system from the very beginning. If users require new skills they should be provided with quality training.

Box 6.3 describes the implementation of an information system that experienced serious problems. It can be used as a case study for identifying and analysing the impact of critical success factors discussed here. For a full report of the project, see the WWW links at the end of the chapter.

BOX 6.3

A HOSPITAL INFORMATION SYSTEM, LIMPOPO PROVINCE, SOUTH AFRICA

This health informatics project involved forty-two hospitals in the Limpopo Province in South Africa. It aimed to improve information use in both clinical and administrative areas by incorporating: master–patient indexes, admissions, discharges, and transfers; order entry and reporting results; departmental systems for laboratory, radiology, and operating theatres; financial management; and hospital performance indicators. Littlejohns et al. (2003) analysed the project and identified the following problems:

- *Infrastructure issues*: for example, a shared electrical circuit resulted in power surges, and network installation was delayed by a concurrent program to upgrade hospitals.
- *Application issues*: introducing too many functions at the one time resulted in some hospitals running the system in a reduced form in parallel with separate pharmacy and laboratory systems.
- *Organisation issues*: poor organisation reduced immediate benefits and caused delays and frustrations for users.

Littlejohns et al. attributed these problems to:

- failure to take into account the professional and social cultures of health care; underestimating the complexity of clinical and managerial processes
- dissonance between expectations of the commissioner, the developer, and users of the system
- long implementation time in the context of fast managerial change
- failure to look for and learn from lessons of past projects.

CONTROLLING IT

If health information systems are to enable more efficient and more effective services, there must be some controls to ensure that information is able to be provided to the appropriate people at the appropriate time in the appropriate format. Developing standards for data transmission and security will facilitate this.

Standards

> Standards provide the bridges to the many islands of electronic patient data so that the data can inexpensively be combined into an electronic medical record (McDonald et al. 1998, p. 213).

The incompatibility of many existing systems is a consequence of the lack of common standards for health care technologies. This continues to be one of the major barriers to increased integration of database and other systems. Standards currently applicable to health informatics were briefly discussed in Chapter 4. Table 6.6 summarises that discussion.

Table 6.6 Standards

Standard	Focus
Vocabularies	Vocabularies are concerned with developing standard terminology to describe symptoms.
Structure and context	These standards provide descriptions of the data elements to be included in documents to be shared.
Messaging	Health information is held in a range of formats in different systems. Messaging standards enable these disparate data sources to be shared between systems by establishing a format and a sequence for data transmission. The HL7 messaging standard is one that is being widely adopted by health services and health software developers and vendors worldwide.
Security standards	Security is a significant issue for developers of health information systems, particularly those that store and transmit patient data. Security standards are designed to protect data from unauthorised or inadvertent access to, or disclosure of, information. Security standards apply to confidentiality, integrity, and availability.

As was noted in Chapter 4, standards are widely, but not universally, accepted. There are a number of groups and organisations involved in the development of standards, and these enjoy varying degrees of acceptance and compliance. Clinical vocabularies, of which there are more than 150, demonstrate the diversity of views, efforts, and degrees of acceptance.

Vocabularies

Vocabularies are concerned with developing standard terminology to describe clinical terms and, as such, they are primarily applicable to electronic health records. Vocabularies are therefore discussed in detail in Chapter 8.

Structure and content standards

While vocabularies provide guidelines for entering clinical data and information into the system, **structure and content standards** should provide a clear description of the data elements to be included in electronic records. This includes:

- establishing essential data elements, such as name, common reference identifier, contact details, temperature, blood pressure (using content headings)
- standardising data structures, such as field length, data type, and acceptable data content for various fields.

Data standards are intended to avoid problems around the ability to use data from other systems because essential elements are missing. By specifying standard lengths and formats for data items, the ease with which data can be shared between systems is greatly enhanced. Table 6.7 is an example of a data standard from the New Zealand Health Information Service website. For more information, check the WWW links at the end of this chapter.

If uniform data structures are to be achieved across all health information systems there are a number of challenges that will need to be met. These include:

- a large investment in non-standard legacy systems
- a large number of owners and users of health systems for whom the ability to share data is not important
- the ever-increasing variety of clinical information structures such as clinical tests, notes, care plans, lists such as for allergies, medications
- the use of image structures for text such as scanned hand-written documents.

Many of the problems of standard data definitions are being addressed by defining standards for metadata, or data about the data. This, together with flexible text mark-up languages such as XML, means that it no longer matters whether a data element such as 'first name' name is allowed 20 or 30 spaces in a record. What does matter is that the receiving system can find out how much space the given name does take and also know where to find it in the data stream being received. Current efforts are focusing on developing interoperability at the level of architectures, rather than detailed data structures.

Messaging standards

Health information is held in a range of formats in different systems. Messaging standards enable these disparate data sources to be shared between systems by establishing a format and a sequence for data transmission. Since following these standards facilitates the exchange of data that people either want or are required to share, there is a great deal of interest in and compliance with these standards. The HL7 messaging

Table 6.7 National Minimum Dataset, New Zealand

Reference	Description	Definition	Format	Valid values	Business rules
	Record type	Code identifying the type of input record	Two characters	HE = Hospital health event HD = Hospital event diagnosis HC = Legal status details	Mandatory
A0012	Health care user (HCU) identifier	The unique identification number assigned to a health care user by the National Health Index (NHI) system	Seven characters	System-generated 3 alpha plus 4 numeric, the last of which is a check digit. Stored as encrypted HCU ID	Mandatory. Must be registered on the NHI before use
A0159	Event type code	Code identifying type of health event	Two characters	Check the event type is on the event type table.	Mandatory. Only one BT event allowed for any NHI number. The presence of some fields depends on the event type, described in detail in Appendix 1. Only the following event types are accepted: BT = Birth event (infants born in reporting hospital). Babies born before mother's admission to hospital or transferred from hospital of birth are recorded as IP. IP = Non-psychiatric inpatient event (include day patients). IM = Psychiatric inpatient event (include day patients). ID = Intended day case.

Source: New Zealand Ministry of Health, 2004.

standard is one that is being widely adopted by health services and health software developers and vendors worldwide. Messaging standards are discussed in more detail in Chapter 7.

Security standards

> Health care providers who are the custodians of confidential information must ensure that information is effectively protected against improper disclosure, modification and use (HB 174-2003, Australia).

The sensitive nature of much health data and information, and the potential for serious consequences of a security breach, have led to the development of specific standards for the security of health data. Technical standards cover areas such as:

- authentication
- access controls
- audit trails
- physical security of technology
- encryption
- system backup and disaster-recovery procedures.

Many developed countries have security standards that deal specifically with health data. Two examples are:

- In Australia, standard HB 174-2003 (Information security management—Implementation guide for the health sector) refers to the general purpose standard for information technology—Code of Practice AS/NZS ISO/IEC 17799:2001—and omits those areas where the general purpose standard is sufficient. Its focus is on the areas of specific concern for the security of health data.
- In the USA, health data is covered by the *Health Insurance Portability and Accountability Act* (HIPAA). The Final Rule adopting HIPAA standards for the security of electronic health information was published in the Federal Register on 20 February 2003. The standards are delineated into either required or addressable implementation specifications.

It is interesting that while a deal of emphasis has been put on standards for keeping health data confidential, the issue of the accuracy of health data managed by large IT systems has not yet been addressed.

SUMMARY

The earliest applications of health information systems in most health services were for administration. While these systems tend to be well accepted, the increasingly integrated information systems environment creates problems for the many ageing systems still in use today.

An information system consists of data, people, technology, procedures, and communication channels that interact to gather, record, process, store, and report information within and between organisations.

In a health care environment, information systems have been classified in terms of their functional area. This describes systems as being used in clinical, administrative, education, research, and other health-related environments. Information systems have been classified according to their purpose. We have transaction processing systems and office automation systems. There are management information systems, decision support systems, executive information systems, and expert systems. Classifying systems in this way gives us an idea of the spread of information systems, across the health care environment, yet does not indicate the different levels and focus of these systems. To achieve this understanding, we can classify systems according to their level of application within the organisation. Thus, systems are described as being used to support strategic, tactical, or operational decision-making.

Early attempts to capture details of health interactions in electronic systems were driven strongly by financial considerations, and the methods used were developed from hospital accounting and billing systems. Today, information systems are used for decision-making, budgeting, and strategic planning. However, while health information systems have been used for many decades, with increasing functionality and integration, the use of these systems varies widely from one health organisation to another.

The complexities of the health care environment create specific challenges for the development of information systems. Early information systems were created to serve a particular purpose within specific departments. The majority of these were developed or purchased independently of one another. As a result, information systems became information silos: locking data within one system, department, or organisation and making it unavailable to other parts of the organisation or service. Today, the existing IT infrastructure in many organisations is a web of interconnected information silos, often running on obsolete hardware and outdated software. Although increasingly unable to meet current information-sharing requirements, they influence, even limit, choices relating to new systems and processes. Nevertheless, for the last decade there has been increasing interest in the development of health information systems that span the enterprise and beyond.

The nature of health and medical information creates particular problems for integrated information systems. Since the object of developing increasingly integrated systems is to facilitate information sharing, we need to overcome the problem of incompatible data. The development of standards is intended to do this.

The introduction of an information system into a health environment can impact on both personal routines and the more formal routines utilised by many within the enterprise. As enterprise systems incorporate more and more clinical routines, this is likely to become an increasingly critical element to be considered.

Effective development of health information systems begins with planning. Strategic planning ensures that the planned systems will fit with the organisation's overall goals and directions. Planning at the project level helps to ensure that the system is functional, meets user needs, and is completed on time.

Approaches to planning include the traditional systems development life cycle, consisting of a series of sequentially completed phases or steps, and rapid applications development, which offers quicker development than the traditional method. This approach, however, is considered unsuitable for unique and/or highly complex programs.

There are a number of critical success factors, which, if addressed, will contribute to the successful development and implementation of a health information system. These include senior management support, utilising a project champion, effective project management, representative team management, end-user participation, and communication.

WWW LINKS

Information strategy

An information strategy for the modern NHS, United Kingdom <http://www.nhsia.nhs.uk/def/
pages/info4health/1.asp>
GP IM & T Strategy Project, NSW Health <http://www.ciap.health.nsw.gov.au/project/gp/downloads/
GP_Strategy%20_Project_Paper_1v1.doc>

Data standards

New Zealand Health Information Service <http://www.nzhis.govt.nz/>

Security standards

General Practice Computing Group, Australia <http://www.gpcg.org/topics/standards.html>
HIPAA, Centers for Medicare and Medicaid, USA <http://www.cms.hhs.gov/hipaa/>

Limpopo Province case study

Littlejohns P., Wyatt, C. & Garvican, L. 2003, 'Evaluating computerised health information systems: hard lessons still to be learnt', *British Medical Journal*, 19 April, no. 320, pp. 800–63 <http://bmj.com>

CRITICAL THINKING

1 Consider ways in which a health organisation that you are familiar with is using information systems at the various levels of management and discuss how they are contributing to better patient outcomes.
2 How might factors discussed in this chapter be influencing the organisation's approach to information systems development?
3 Draw a simple data flow diagram for one small section of the organisation.
4 What might be critical strategic, tactical, and operational success factors for the LASCAD system (discussed in Chapter 2) and the Limpopo project?
5 What type of planning was used for the Limpopo project? Was there an approach that might have been more effective? Use this approach to write a plan for the project.

CHAPTER 7

E-HEALTH

OVERVIEW

The term 'e-health' sounds so twenty-first century, conjuring up images of specialist clinicians using the latest communication, information, and robotics technologies to operate on patients on the other side of the world; of patients logging onto the Internet to find the latest information about a health issue, or to consult their online physician; of clinicians holding a case conference with colleagues around the world.

These phenomena have occurred, but e-health is still in its infancy. Many initiatives are still at the project stage and programs are only just beginning to be absorbed into mainstream health care. There are many issues to be resolved. Thus, while it is widely believed that the use of e-health-enabled services will change health care delivery, the nature of the changes is not yet clear. What is clear, however, is that any change must be a result of the way in which health professionals, consumers, administrators, and managers adopt, shape, and use e-health. People must drive the technology, rather than the technology driving people.

OBJECTIVES

At the completion of this chapter, you should be able to:
- discuss perceptions of telemedicine, telehealth, and e-health
- describe current health care applications coming under the umbrella of e-health
- discuss issues to be considered when planning and implementing an e-health service or application
- discuss measures to facilitate involvement of the e-health consumer in his or her own health care.

CONCEPTS AND TERMS

Telemedicine
E-health
Telehealth

INTRODUCTION

This chapter explores the emerging phenomenon known as e-health. It begins by identifying the drivers, scope, and applications of e-health. Key player perspectives, instrumental in shaping e-health services, are explored and discussed. Issues and challenges to
be dealt with when developing and implementing such programs are also considered.

Although the term 'e-health' is widely used, the terms 'e-health-enabled services'
and 'telehealth-enabled services' are used occasionally in the chapter to reinforce that
technology is a *tool* to enable the delivery of health services. This is consistent with the
socio-technical perspective of health informatics.

USING E-HEALTH

The ideal e-health system

> Borderless. Seamless. Accessible in all reaches of the country. Delivering fast, accurate
> diagnosis and treatment. A system where health care providers are equipped to focus on
> prevention and evidence-based treatment. Where all points of care (such as homes,
> schools, family practitioners, community clinics and hospitals) are linked. Free from red
> tape and wasteful duplication. Offering individuals the tools to take control over their
> own health. Where the privacy, security and confidentiality of personal health informa-
> tion are respected (Health Canada 2000, p. 1).

Here we have an ideal health system that benefits all and disadvantages no one. But is
this possible?

An ideal system would require a delicate balancing act. Consider, for example, the
following questions:

- Is there a point when a focus on prevention leads to inadequate resources for acute
  care?
- When *do* guidelines, policies, and procedures to ensure quality standards become
  red tape?
- When might consumers' control over their own health care become compromised
  through lack of knowledge?
- Is there a point when the consumer's right to privacy and confidentiality conflicts
  with the health care provider's requirement for information to provide safe care?

In seeking to answer questions such as these, it quickly becomes clear that an 'ideal'
system from one perspective may be less than ideal from another. When developing
e-health-enabled services, we need to be aware of the different perspectives and the key
players that are their source. Key players may include:

- *Consumers*: patients and their families, support and advocacy groups, local communities
- *Health care providers*: health professionals and their representative organisations
- *Health care managers*: hospitals, public, and private health services

- *Health care funders*: State and federal governments, and health insurance organisations, among others
- *E-health businesses*: information and telecommunications companies and commercial health-related businesses trading online
- *Academic and other institutions*: those engaged in research and development.

Each group will have a different view of the potential benefits and issues. Box 7.1 explores some of these different views.

BOX 7.1 STAKEHOLDER PERCEPTIONS OF E-HEALTH

Health care managers and funders may focus on cost savings and increased efficiencies, while consumers may be concerned about the location of services and waiting times. Within each broad group of key stakeholders there will be subgroups with different points of view. The health care manager group might include administrators who view e-health as offering increased business efficiency, and public health officials who view e-health as a means of monitoring and managing public health. Among providers, rural health practitioners may view the potential of e-health primarily in terms of increased and speedier access to test results and specialist services, while specialists in large city hospitals may view the same services as creating extra demands on already limited time.

These different views may conflict with each other and key stakeholders will have different levels of power and influence in presenting their views. As a consequence, some stakeholders may (albeit inadvertently) shape services in a way that significantly disadvantages other groups. While the system we arrive at will no doubt be an attempt to balance the interests of all participants, it will be an ideal system for none.

What are we talking about?

Because of the rapidly changing environment of information technology, definitions change quickly (Rider 2002, p. 1).

The terms 'e-health', 'telehealth', and 'telemedicine' are all used to describe the use of videoconferencing, the Internet, and other communications technology (including the telephone) in the delivery of health care services, with the emphasis being on the means of communication. As with other aspects of health informatics, the terms are not used consistently. Fluid terminology is to be expected in an emerging discipline where key concepts are still being defined, rapidly evolving technology produces new terms to differentiate each new development, and territorial differences often shape the discussion. An historical perspective offers some insight into how the various terms evolved and are used.

The first 'telemedicine' services date back to the early twentieth century. An example is the Australian Royal Flying Doctor Service, organised in the late 1920s by John Flynn. This service used a pedal wireless and aircraft to establish a system of regular long-distance medical consultations, with doctors being flown to patients in emergencies.

The services that are generally thought of as telemedicine emerged during the 1950s and 1960s. These early services used broadcast television technologies to send images and data: 'Audio and visual data were not integrated with other clinical data, stored or otherwise available. Telecommunications was merely a mode of transporting signals, in which the coordination of multiple complex signals was costly, cumbersome, and not sufficiently reliable for most clinical applications' (Bashshur & Shannon 2002, p. 1). Box 7.2 describes some early telemedicine projects.

BOX 7.2

EARLY TELEMEDICINE PROJECTS

Nebraska Medical Center

In 1964, a two-way, closed-circuit television link was established between the Nebraska Psychiatric Institute and Norfolk State Hospital, 112 miles away. It was used for education, and consultations between specialists and general practitioners. In 1971, the Center was linked with the Omaha Veterans Administration Hospital and veterans affairs facilities in two other towns.

Space Technology Applied to Rural Papago Advanced Health Care (STARPAHC)

The STARPAHC project ran from 1972 to 1975. Its goals were to provide health care to astronauts in space and to provide general medical care to the Papago Reservation. A van staffed by American Indian paramedics carried a variety of medical instruments including electrocardiograph and x-ray. This was linked to the two hospitals by a two-way microwave telemedicine and audio transmission.

North-West Telemedicine Project

This project was set up in 1984 in Australia to pilot test a government satellite communications network (the Q-Network). The project goals were to provide health care to people in five remote towns south of the Gulf of Carpentaria. The Q-Network consisted of twenty two-way earth stations and twenty one-way (television receivers only) earth stations. The hub of the network was the Mount Isa Base Hospital. All sites were supplied with a conference telephone, fax, and freeze-frame transceivers. Evaluation for the project showed that the technology did improve the health care of these remote residents (Brown 1995).

Early applications often focused on clinical services or clinical education and were thus referred to as telemedicine. Quite a few telemedicine projects were established in this period, mostly in isolation, and not as part of the overall strategic development of a health service.

Most projects did not survive beyond their initial funding period. Of those that did, 'high costs, limitations of the technology and the inherent conservatism within both the medical profession and wider community resulted in telemedicine remaining on the periphery rather than being absorbed into mainstream health care' (McDonald et al. 1998, p. 14).

During the early 1990s, rapid advances in telecommunications technology saw mainstream interest in telemedicine increase. Bashshur and Shannon (2002, p. 1) identify key developments as the introduction of integrated service digital networks (ISDN), digital telecommunications channels, and protocols. These greatly enhanced the quality and capability of transmissions. Services expanded beyond clinical consultation and clinical information transfer to include a range of professional and community education, as well as administration. The term 'telehealth' began to be used to describe the broader applications, while 'telemedicine' continued to be used to describe clinical services. Telemedicine was thus viewed by many as a subset of telehealth.

The late 1990s signalled the beginnings of what is generally referred to as e-health. Converging information and communications technology and the development of protocols and standards such as transmission control protocol (TCP) Internet protocol (IP), simple mail transfer protocol (SMTP), and hypertext mark-up language (HTML) created the means to communicate and exchange information quickly and easily anywhere in the world.

Health services began to explore the potential of the Internet for delivery of information and services both at a distance and within an immediate community, such as a hospital or medical practice. Today, e-health activity is expanding rapidly to encompass many areas of health research, care, and education. Some examples are discussed later in the chapter.

The use of videoconferencing also continues to expand. While these services may be directed towards rural, remote, and housebound individuals, videoconferencing is also used to facilitate communication in other environments, such as between health professionals in large hospitals, or between facilities in city and urban environments.

E-health or telehealth?

Distinctions between telehealth and e-health have been made on the basis of:

- *Distance*: Telehealth is generally the term of choice when distance is a critical factor. It can, however, be difficult to ascertain when distance becomes 'critical'.
- *Technology*: Telehealth is largely non-Internet-based, and characterised by point-to-point and dial-up information exchange. E-health is Internet-based and therefore much more widely accessible (Maheu 2000). These distinctions are becoming increasingly blurred with the convergence of communications and information technology (such as Internet telephony and IP videoconferencing).

- *Nature of the transmission*: Telehealth focuses on voice and video, e-health on digital data transmission.
- *Model of service delivery*: Telehealth follows the top-down model of traditional health care delivery, with the professional as expert. E-health on the other hand, with its extensive use of the Internet, allows people access to information and knowledge formerly the province of the expert (Maheu 2000).

Another way of distinguishing between types of services is on the basis of their location and scope. On the one hand, there are services typically available, managed, and controlled within health care systems, while on the other hand, there are those available outside these formal systems. Services within health care systems include point-to-point, dial-up transmissions, and Internet-based applications. These programs reside within, and are administered by, health systems. Many of the issues they face are typical organisation issues around quality of service, equity of access, acceptance by professionals and consumers, efficiency, cost and reliability of equipment, and privacy, legal, and ethical constraints.

Services outside formal health systems operate in a broader arena, where commercial and business interests, community groups, and individuals predominantly use the Internet to offer activities, information, and services. These are much wider in scope, much less coordinated, and much less controlled than those offered by traditional service systems. This broad field of activity brings to the fore different issues for health care systems, governments, and the community. These issues revolve around the quality, reliability, and safety of information, goods, and services. Many are beyond the ability of the health care system to control, yet may have a significant impact on that system. Consumer use of the Internet to gather information, for example, is changing relationships with health professionals, who have a limited ability to influence consumer behaviour, but do need to respond to it.

Thus, services can be distinguished on the basis of the issues they create.

Drivers of e-health

> The first use of the word [e-health] may be traced back to industry leaders and marketing staff...(Wachter 2002, p. 1).

E-health has evolved in response to social, political, economic, and technological drivers both within health care systems and in the wider society. These drivers include:

- urbanisation and the decline of rural communities' equity of access
- an ageing population
- technology, market forces, and the rise of the health consumer.

Urbanisation and the decline of rural communities' equity of access

Since the earliest use of telehealth and e-health, a key driver has been the need to provide or maintain health care services to remote or isolated areas. This has become increasingly significant in recent years with declining rural populations and increasing concern about service levels in the rural and remote areas. At the same time, health costs continue to rise. Governments are funding e-health projects in the hope of increasing efficiency while also improving health outcomes. Box 7. 3 typifies this.

BOX 7.3

E-HEALTH FOR RURAL COMMUNITIES

Canada
The health system faces certain unique challenges that include care delivery to a significant portion of the population, distributed sparsely across a landmass of 10 million square kilometres, in areas of extreme climactic conditions. The promise of e-health lies in the manner and degree to which it can mitigate or resolve these challenges (Alvarez 2002).

Australia
All states are active in the area of telehealth, expanding the number of services in rural and remote areas, as well as innovative applications of the technology. Telehealth services have been shown to improve access to care, promote greater integration of remote health services, and improve support for staff in rural and remote areas (AHMAC 2003).

Table 7.1 illustrates that this is not simply talk. Governments and health systems are making extensive use of e-health, particularly telehealth, in their efforts to reduce inequities of access due to distance and geography.

Table 7.1 Telehealth activity according to accessibility/remoteness of hospitals

	Highly accessible	Accessible accessible	Moderately Remote	Remote	Very remote	Total
No telehealth	191 (65%)	70 (48%)	22 (31%)	3 (12%)	3 (10%)	289 (51%)
Some telehealth	103 (35%)	76 (52%)	48 (69%)	21 (88%)	27 (90%)	275 (49%)
Total	294 (100%)	146 (100%)	70 (100%)	24 (100%)	30 (100%)	564 (100%)

Source: Wootton et al. 2003

The research of Wootton et al. (2003) found a clear linear trend of increasing remoteness associated with increased involvement in telehealth activity.

An ageing population

The Australian Bureau of Statistics (ABS) predicts that 'as the youngest of the baby-boom generation turns 65 in 2031, the median age of the population is projected to reach between 42–43 years, and the proportion of the population aged 65 and over is projected to reach between 21 and 22 per cent' (2002).

The ageing population is causing concern among consumers and health care providers alike. It is anticipated by some that an ageing population will result in increased demand and costs for health services. An alternative view is that the high costs of health care for the elderly are principally related to medical management of the end of life, and that these end of life costs will not necessarily be greater in an older population. E-health offers the potential to maintain the health status of older people, manage chronic conditions with minimal attendance at health care facilities, and support frailer older people for longer in their own homes.

Technology, market forces, and the rise of the health consumer

Technology companies encouraged and supported many early telemedicine, telehealth, and e-health programs. They 'saw the health care sector as a particularly attractive industry that will benefit from web-based technologies because of its enormous size, inefficiency and information intensity' (Coiera 1997, p. 243). This facilitated the development of e-health within the health care system. The influence of different perspectives on health informatics was discussed in Chapter 2. E-health is an area where the commercial perspective can be seen to have been particularly influential.

> The trend in the USA is for large IT companies such as Intel and Microsoft to merge with health online companies, to form new companies exploiting the capabilities of online communication...[T]he Australian Government and industry need to continue to work together to ensure that high technology research and development leads to the rapid commercialisation of e-health technologies. Both parties also need to work together to grow Australian-based technology companies in this area (Mitchell & Associates 1999, pp. 4–5).

Health consumers are also driving e-health. In recent years, consumers with access to the Internet have become proactive not only in their health and medical care, but also in their choice of health professionals. They have become consumers, rather than patients.

The link between drivers and key players

Drivers often reflect the needs, wants, and influence of key players. While emerging technology is considered to be a driver of e-health, it may well be the need for telecommunications and information technology companies to create markets and produce profits that is actually driving the use of the technology in health care. So too with the ageing population. It may not be the ageing population itself that is the driver, but the need for governments and health services to provide adequate, cost-efficient, and accessible health care that is driving the development of e-health.

Applications of e-health

E-health-enabled services are many and varied, including clinical, education, administrative, research, and commercial activities. The technology used to conduct these activities is equally diverse, and continues to expand. The following is a brief overview of the range of activities and services falling under the umbrella of e-health.

Clinical activities

Within health care organisations, the range of teleservices, including telepsychiatry, teleradiology, telecardiology, and telepaediatrics, attests to the long history of using videoconferencing for direct consultation and exchange of clinical information. While many of these services use analog transmissions for quality reasons, digital transmissions are being increasingly used for clinical services, including the transmission of documents and images. Advances in technology are also seeing previously unsuited activities become part of the e-health environment. Examples include:

- Digital cameras and mobile phones with digital photography capabilities, for example, are enabling clinical consultations for skin conditions, an area previously excluded due to poor visual quality of the images.
- An AIDS management program in South Africa uses mobile phone SMS messages to monitor compliance with drug therapy in remote communities.
- Wireless technology is enabling health professionals to access information and communicate from diverse locations, thereby increasing the scope and flexibility of e-health services.

Beyond health care organisations, the use of the Internet for direct clinical consultations has been limited, but is increasing. Medical groups and individual professionals are using the Internet to offer advice and, increasingly, to offer direct consultations. Commercial enterprises are using the Internet to sell medications, alternative therapies, books, and other health-related goods and services. Yet, as Yellowlees observes, 'this is cowboy country at present' (2000, p. 41). It is largely unmonitored and uncontrolled. A significant issue in this area of e-health is the quality of these services, particularly if they are offered outside the established health care system and, as is frequently the case, from an overseas location.

Information

The role of health informatics in information retrieval was discussed in Chapter 2, and a number of examples were given. The Internet is becoming a primary information-retrieval tool for health professionals and consumers alike. Health professionals are using the Internet to access and exchange information with peers locally and around the world. Consumers are accessing information primarily via the many Internet information sites, subject-specific chat rooms, and mailing lists. Health care organisations, and commercial, community, and special interest groups are acknowledging this trend by using the Internet to disseminate information. The quality of the information accessed by consumers is seen as an issue by many health departments and professionals.

Education

A wide range of professional development programs and community education programs are utilising e-health technologies. Programs range from tertiary-level formal courses to informal short courses and discussion groups. The Internet lends itself particularly to education for the complex, geographically, and professionally diverse health care community, since it provides access to comprehensive resources, and opportunities for synchronous and asynchronous communication.

BOX 7.4 EXAMPLES OF E-HEALTH EDUCATION ACTIVITIES

- A tele-otology course for primary care providers: a multi-media course for primary care providers, incorporating material about ear anatomy and physiology, ear disease, video-otoscopy, and telemedicine software. The program included a computer-based course followed by a practical one- or two-day course.
- A web-based e-learning tool for teaching nursing skills, using educational material from a hospital-based nursing fair. A manager function tracks skill certification and continuing education contact hours. The content can be delivered over the Internet and through firewalls using Windows Media Player version 9.

Health service intranets and extranets

Health services are using intranets to improve communication and the flow of information within their organisation. Intranets are also becoming integral to the information systems used to expedite the daily activities of organisations. Extranets connecting the health care organisation to its partners are also becoming increasingly common.

Measuring success

Evaluation of programs and services can provide evidence of the value of e-health, and inform more effective future planning and development. At present, however, useful information from evaluation is quite limited. One reason for this is the broad range of services and activities falling under the umbrella of e-health. These diverse programs differ in focus, technology used, target group, goals, and outcomes. This makes it difficult to draw any general conclusions from available research and evaluation (Dillon & Loermans 2003).

The very newness of many services is another factor limiting the usefulness of research. Many services have not been established long enough for the evaluation cycle to be completed. Therefore, most available research focuses on the longer-established telemedicine and telehealth programs. Since many of these are short-term pilot or proof-of-concept programs, evaluations often focus on describing services, measuring hits to websites, or using other descriptive, rather than analytical, evaluation criteria.

Identifying analytical criteria presents a further difficulty. A number of different criteria may be used to evaluate e-health programs and services. These include safety, efficacy, cost effectiveness, clinical utility, and user satisfaction. Unfortunately, as Coiera (2004, p. 267) notes, 'most evaluations have tended to focus on user satisfaction, rather than attempting to measure system effects in a quantitative way. This makes generalising about the value of e-health difficult'. In support of this, KPMG Consulting (1999) identified the following issues relating to the evaluation of telehealth:

- few generalisable studies
- very limited discussion of evaluation design and methods used
- very little long-term follow-up data collection
- the focus on acceptability and satisfaction of the service provider and the patient/client, but no standard tools to measure these aspects
- little consistency in the measurement of costs
- highly application-dependent measures of clinical effectiveness and that are difficult to generalise.

It should be noted that these shortcomings are not exclusive to telehealth, but apply to evaluations of many health informatics systems and applications, including information systems and the broad area of e-health today.

There is some research that might provide insights into the effectiveness and efficiency of e-health and telehealth services. Partly as a consequence of the problems discussed above, however, this research has produced mixed findings. Box 7.5 lists some findings relating to e-health and telehealth.

BOX 7.5 MIXED EVALUATION RESULTS

Telehealth-enabled services are more readily adopted by health professionals and consumers in hub sites located in rural areas than by specialist clinicians in urban spoke sites...Not being able to touch the patient, and the extra time involved in telehealth consults, have been found to influence clinician response (Moulton et al. 2002).

Consumers are very willing to adopt the Internet as a tool for seeking information and support (Yellowlees 2000).

Home monitoring services are received more positively by some consumers and professionals than others (Coiera 2004, McGee 2004, Peisner 2004).

These findings suggest that e-health technologies are more suitable for some consumers and health professionals, some environments and some services but not others. To facilitate the effective use of e-health, it is therefore necessary to ensure that the services provided are appropriate. This means focusing on the problems to be resolved, rather than the technology to be used.

ENABLING E-HEALTH SERVICES

The perfusion of high quality information technology into the heart of health care should lead to radical redesign (Smith 2004b, p. 328).

To facilitate the success of e-health programs, planning must take into account key stakeholder perspectives, include an analysis of the organisational and cultural aspects, and consider the technical issues.

Planning

The development and implementation of e-health is a managed process. Very small projects—such as a static web page for a small community centre, or a series of education sessions using existing videoconferencing equipment may require relatively simple planning involving one or two people and a checklist of things to do. A large project, such as an interactive hospital website offering online information, appointment bookings, test results, and other information, or the establishment of a home monitoring system for frail elderly people, will require the involvement of many more people and a significant budget. Different types of projects will also require different technology and expertise. The planning process was introduced in Chapter 4. Table 7.2 summarises this process.

Table 7.2 Summary of planning process

Planning phase	Purpose and activities
Business case	Documents the costs, benefits, and risks inherent in a project; assesses fit between organisational goals and project
Project definition	Identifies problem; scopes proposed solution; specifies outputs and intended outcomes; lists benefits to key players; outlines resources required
Planning	Participative process: evolves and changes as the project progresses; may be reviewed, revised, and expanded after input from the project team and key players, after a review of available resources or at any other time through the life of the project
Control and monitoring	As each stage is completed, the project team evaluates both the outcome of that phase, and the way it was achieved. Modifications to the plan may be made
Outcomes realisation	Ensure that work practices are modified appropriately to take full advantage of the opportunities and changes delivered by the project

The initial phases of planning will seek to identify:

- the problem to be resolved by the proposed system
- who the system is intended to serve
- what services are expected to be provided
- balance between capacity and demand: often expectations, or demands, will outweigh the capacity of the service to provide them
- tradeoffs: needs and wants of key players may well conflict.

In dealing with these points, the views of the large number of disparate interest groups, each with its own agenda, will need to be considered.

Key player perspectives

The support of a number of these groups, or key players, will impact on an e-health program or service. In this process, key players range from those who shape policy and make funding decisions at a strategic level, to those who ensure that a service will be successful by using it. Strategic players include governments and large commercial organisations that can create a positive climate for e-health by providing the necessary funding, infrastructure, software, and hardware. Other strategic players are the policy makers and management responsible for strategic planning within health care organisations. Key players at the tactical and operational level include middle management, who coordinate the implementation of e-health services, and health care professionals, ICT professionals, administrative and support staff, and consumers, who implement, maintain, and use the services on a day-to-day basis.

The views of key players will colour their ideas about the appropriate structure, technology, and service mix for e-health services. Chapter 2 identified a number of different views or perspectives, including technology, administrator, commercial, consumer, and clinical. Key players may hold any one or combination of these perspectives. They may also change their perspective over time or in different circumstances.

Government

Governments establish policies and provide many of the resources to enable health care organisations to implement e-health services, particularly where health care is partially or fully resourced from public funds. A supportive government facilitates the growth of e-health. Australia is an example of a country with supportive government. Box 7.6 illustrates this.

Governments also influence e-health by their willingness to modify existing procedures and guidelines to accommodate services. The issue of reimbursement for services illustrates this. Many health care providers have experienced difficulty in obtaining reimbursement for telehealth e-health consultations, as these fall outside existing guidelines. This may influence the willingness of health professionals to use the services: 'The greatest challenge in e-health right now is reimbursement...as long as doctors and hospitals are unsure about whether they'll get paid...the services won't reach their full potential' (McGee 2004). Reimbursement issues are being addressed, with some services such as telepsychiatry now approved for reimbursement. However, the

BOX 7.6

AUSTRALIAN GOVERNMENT SUPPORT FOR E-HEALTH

In 1998, Australian Health Ministers established the National Health Information Management Advisory Council (NHIMAC). The Council has developed Health*Online*, a detailed action plan aimed at improving health care through the application of information technology. In June 1999, the Australian Government introduced the Practice Incentive Payments (PIP) scheme to stimulate the uptake of computers in Australian general practice. In August 2002, 90 per cent of general practitioners were using electronic prescribing and 89 per cent had the capacity for electronic data interchange. This compares with 51 per cent and 68 per cent respectively in August 1999. The Australian Government has been active in ensuring that the telecommunications infrastructure is extended across the country, including to rural and remote areas, for e-health both within the health care system and in the wider e-health environment. The Australian Government seeks to incorporate the views of all key players in its strategic initiatives.

fact that psychiatric services were one of the pioneers of telehealth indicates the gap between developments in technology and the many social, legal, and economic issues needing to be addressed.

Issues around state–federal jurisdiction are another example. Legislation relating to the delivery of services may vary from state to state, and between state and federal governments. Since e-health cuts across boundaries, states may need to cooperate to adjust legislation accordingly: 'Because health care is regulated along State lines and because telemedicine is a technology that is innately disrespectful of conventional borders, it is inevitable that if and when a telemedicine service crosses a State or Territorial border or involves a "multi-jurisdictional" component, difficult policy, regulatory and legal questions will arise' (Milstein 1999, p. 4). Issues relate to cross-border consultations (in which State is the doctor practising medicine?), defining the 'practice of medicine', and identifying how regulators might need to distinguish between the various service-delivery options available through e-health. For a more detailed discussion see the WWW links at the end of the chapter.

Suppliers

> Hundreds of businesses have sprouted up to save health care from its much-lamented technological ineptitude (Russell 2000, p. 1).

Since suppliers of infrastructure, software, hardware, and expertise are operating businesses, they will adopt a commercial perspective towards e-health. As the bulk of the goods and services they offer are technology based, their perspective is also technological. This may be at odds with views of other key players. Yet suppliers can have a strategic impact. The willingness of telecommunications companies to invest in the relevant infrastructure, and to make it available at an affordable price, is crucial to the development of e-health. The willingness or capacity of developers and vendors of hardware, software, and expertise to tailor their products to service needs, and to offer reliable, high quality goods and services will impact on the willingness of management, health professionals, and consumers to use e-health services.

Health care organisations

Senior management within health care organisations also set strategic directions that shape e-health services. Health care organisations seek to provide high quality, efficient services to the greatest number of consumers at the lowest cost. For private health care organisations, a profit margin will also be part of the equation. Health organisations have finite resources and many demands for these. Funding for e-health services will often be at the expense of other services. The views of senior management will set parameters around the nature, scope, and focus of e-health programs.

Dominant discourses or perspectives will shape projects. A focus on efficiency, technology, or quality care will produce different issues and different outcomes. For example, electronic home monitoring is seen as more efficient use of resources, since the health professional need only visit when needed. There is a risk, however, that this administrator perspective may overshadow the views of health professionals and consumers, with the consequence that inappropriate use of home monitoring will lead to a reduction in justifiable home visits. This may, in turn result in an increase in social isolation, particularly among older patients (McGee 2004).

Health professionals

Health professional organisations, particularly peak bodies, can have a strategic impact on e-health. These bodies can endorse e-health by supporting initiatives, offering relevant education, and accrediting related activities.

Individual health professionals have a significant influence at the day-to-day levels of e-health. The large and diverse group known as health professionals contains many smaller groups of key players. These groupings may fall along professional lines, but may also cut across these and form around service type or geographical location. Responses and views of health professionals must therefore be viewed as contextual. They will vary depending on time, place, and type of service.

Health professionals are concerned with providing high quality care for their patients. They will therefore view e-health in terms of its relevance to, and effectiveness in furthering this goal. Limited physical contact and interaction, one-to-one personal care, unreliable technology, and time involved setting up consultations are the types of issues that have been found to influence health professionals (Tanriverdi & Iacono 1999, McGee 2004, Moulton 2004). As many of these assessments are subjective, services may be perceived as relevant and effective by some professionals, but not by others. For example, telehealth at a remote site improves access to many specialist services and professional resources previously available on a limited basis and usually involving travel, while in a hub site the health professional provides the service regardless and usually it is the patient who travels. In the former environment, telehealth is more likely to be perceived as relevant and effective than it is in the latter.

Consumers

> The first generation of e-patients has arrived (Ferguson & Frydman 2004).

Consumers view e-health from the perspective of equity of access and quality of service. Their views appear to be influenced by issues around the ability to access services as well as, or better than, they did previously, on the quality of the interaction, information and/or advice, including the quality of the transmission, and costs or cost savings (McGee 2004, Moulton 2004, Peisner 2004).

Consumers choose whether or not to adopt the available services. This is often a limited option, although the increasing availability of advice, information, and services on the Internet is enhancing consumers' ability to exercise this option. These developments are changing the traditional health professional–consumer relationship: 'The relationship of the twenty-first century will be one of mutual participation. It implies equality, trust and collaboration, with both parties needing and depending on the other's input' (Yellowlees 2000, p. 104).

Balancing key player perspectives

Planning can be so helpful. If done effectively, planning will help to ensure that key player perspectives have been considered and, where possible, incorporated into the project or service. Having said this, the reality is usually that one or two key player perspectives dominate, while others are marginalised.

Table 7.3 Project definition document

Definition issue	Blue Skies professional education project
Problem	Provision of timely professional development to rural health care nurses
Outputs	An education and information website accessible from remote locations Seminars and case discussions via teleconference
Intended outcomes	More informed nursing staff
Benefits to key players	More efficient use of professional development resources Increased retention of rural health care nurses Enhanced quality of care to consumers
Resources required	Establishment Ongoing: professional information, technology maintenance, help desk

The preparation of the business case will enable the proposed program or service to be linked to the strategic goals of the organisation. Significant projects or services may also be linked to the broader health environment. This might include reference to the goals and objectives of government and other strategic players, demographic and consumer trends. As Table 7.3 shows, project definition can ensure a problem-solving focus rather than a technology focus.

Participative planning will facilitate the involvement of key players, including users of the system. This will ensure that issues around access, usability, workflows and routines, and user satisfaction are all addressed.

Cultural and organisational issues: change management

> Some doctors and caregivers also resist e-health initiatives, particularly when it involves changes in workflow and culture (McGee 2004).

Health professionals, like most of us, will more willingly adopt a change such as the introduction of e-health-enabled services, if it is clearly an improvement on the existing ways of doing things. Often this improvement is not clear, at least initially, and sometimes the change is not an improvement.

New technologies often disrupt traditional work routines, workflow, and work relationships. The location of equipment, the need to consult with others, the protocols involved, and the need to enter and access information in a timely manner may all have an impact. Clinician–consumer interaction may suffer: 'When using e-health technology, particularly where they had received only minimal training, health professionals were often preoccupied with the computer, rather than focused on their patient' (Greatbatch et al. 2001). Greatbatch et al. found that this did not diminish as clinicians became more familiar with the equipment.

Since e-health technologies are designed for collaboration and information sharing, health professionals are able to interact with one another in ways not previously explored. While this clearly offers opportunities for enhanced services, the issue of status, power, and authority (not to mention issues such as ownership of, and responsibility for, medical records) may become a problem for some professionals.

The response of health professionals to the introduction of e-health will be partly shaped by the organisational context within which they operate. Organisation theory suggests that organisations differ in their willingness or ability to change. The traditional, hierarchical organisation, which characterises many of today's health care services, is generally perceived as more resistant to change than the flatter, more teamwork-oriented structures adopted by some services in recent years. Yet both types of organisations have successfully implemented e-health services. This suggests that change and resistance to change may be context dependent and different strategies will be appropriate for different enterprise structures (Briggs 2001, Kinyon 2003): 'Planning for the introduction of online health programs in organisations needs to include strategies compatible with the dominant characteristics of that organisation' (Walker & Whetton 2002, p. 74).

Technical Matters

Chapter 4 discussed the basics of networking. This chapter draws on that discussion as it relates to e-health.

Connectivity: linking people

To benefit from e-health, consumers must have the capability to access it. Services offered online are intended to increase access. Yet inadequate connectivity may in fact reduce access. The type of connections used will impact on the efficiency and quality of the service provided. The connections used must be able to support and manage the type of service to be provided and the data to be transmitted. Box 7.7 illustrates this.

BOX 7.7

CONNECTIVITY CONSIDERATIONS

Bandwidth

Bandwidth must be high enough to enable the intended types and volume of data to be transmitted quickly and reliably. The more data there is to send, the fatter the 'pipe' must be. The pipe needs to be considerably fatter in order to deliver a high-resolution digital image such as an X-ray, compared with a text-based report, in the same time. It is therefore important to know the type of files a network is intended to handle, and whether the transmission needs to be in real time. It is important for IP video transmissions to be received in real time, or very close to it, and occasional lost 'packets' of information can have a marked impact on the quality of the picture. On the other hand, it is acceptable for Picture Archiving Communications Systems (PACS) images from a radiology procedure to be delivered over a period of many minutes, with the entire image viewable when transmission is complete.

Wireless

Wireless technology uses radio signals, not hardwired systems, to transmit data. Wireless technology enables mobile caregivers, such as nurses and physicians, to have access to data wherever and whenever it is needed, and can also be used to provide network connections in areas where it would be difficult or expensive to install cable or fibre. The general packet radio service (GPRS) allows communication to remote users across global system for mobile (GSM) phone networks, providing a wireless wide area network (WAN) for health workers away from cabled sites. Although wireless can be very convenient, there are still issues relating to security.

These technology issues are within the area of expertise of information and computing professionals. The health informatics professional needs to be aware of the issues without being an expert.

Interface: sharing data and information

In 1987, an organisation known as Health Level 7 (HL7) was formed with the goal of providing flexible, cost-effective approaches, standards, guidelines, methodologies, and related services for interoperability between health care information systems (HL7 2004).

Interface problems relate to computers and users being able to format data and define and share the meaning of the information thus created. This is being achieved through the development of standards such as HL7, a messaging protocol specifically developed to enable the exchange of information in the clinical and health administration domains. The term HL7 refers to the seventh layer of the ISO network communications model. This is the application layer, which means that HL7 applies to the formatting or structure of information but does not specify the technical details of how the network passes information from one system to another. HL7 is an accepted international standard, with affiliates in a number of countries including Australia. A number of HL7 standards and protocols have been released and are being applied, while new protocols are currently being developed. Table 7.4, a table of abstracts for each of the current American National Standards Institute (ANSI) HL7 standards, provides some idea of the areas covered by HL7.

A look at the Australian, Canadian, New Zealand, and the United Kingdom HL7 websites indicates vigorous debate and active input into the HL7 standards and provides hope for at least one universal worldwide standard for health care data. See the WWW links at the end of the chapter for these sites.

Extensible Markup Language (XML)

XML is a formal recommendation of the World Wide Web Consortium (W3C), an international group that aims to develop interoperable technologies (specifications, guidelines, software, and tools) to enable exploitation of the Web to its fullest potential. XML is used to code format and content in a way that allows information to be exchanged across diverse hardware, operating systems, and applications. Information formatted in XML can be exchanged across platforms, languages, and applications, and can be used with a wide range of development tools and utilities.

Most databases were originally designed to process and store only the type of data that fits neatly into rows and columns. This was a limitation to the integration of health information systems, since much of the health data to be stored exists as image, video, or other non-text data formats. XML can be extended to contain any imaginable data type, from classical data such as text and numbers, or multimedia objects such as sounds, to active formats such as Java applets or ActiveX components.

In health informatics, XML is being used to develop data structures and messages that can be accessed and exchanged via the Internet.

Table 7.4 HL7 standards

Standard	Title	Abstract
ANSI/HL7 Arden V2.1-2002	Health Level Seven Arden Syntax for Medical Logic Systems, Version 2.1	The principal new feature of this version of the standard is the augmentation of the WRITE statement with a structured message.
ANSI/HL7 CDA R1.0-2000	The HL7 Version 3 Standard: Clinical Data Architecture, Release 1.0	The HL7 Clinical Document Architecture defines an XML architecture for the exchange of clinical documents. The encoding is based on XML DTDs included in the specification and its semantics are defined using the HL7 RIM (Reference Information Model) and HL7 registered coded vocabularies.
ANSI/HL7 CMS V1.4-2002	HL7 Context Management Specification, Version 1.4	The Health Level Seven Context Management Specification is a standard for visually integrating independently developed health care application programs for concurrent use by a single user.
ANSI/HL7 V2.4-2000	Health Level Seven Standard Version 2.4 Application Protocol for Electronic Data Exchange in Health Care	Includes minor enhancements and fixes, as well as new messages for the master patient index (MPI), a chapter for lab automation messages, and a new chapter for messages pertaining to personnel management. Query messages have been broken out into a separate chapter, and network management messages have been moved into a normative chapter.

Source: compiled from the American National Standards Institute 2004

MANAGING E-HEALTH

This final section considers security issues necessary to enable the safe and effective delivery of health services. It also considers the informed consumer, who is increasingly influential in the e-health arena.

Security

Issues include:

- Protecting networks
- Protecting users: email attacks
- Protecting users: Internet attacks

Protecting networks

E-health applications send a range of data across various types of communication lines. While cryptography can help to ensure the confidentiality of the data, it does not protect the communication channels or networks themselves.

Communication channels can be viewed in terms of those where the links and users are trusted and those that are not. Many e-health applications create connections between trusted and less trusted networks as, for example, a connection between a private provider and a public provider. The security obligations and policies for the two networks will probably differ and interactions between the two will need to be checked to ensure that traffic entering one network from the other conforms to the policies of that network. This is particularly true when connections are made to the Internet, which must be viewed as completely untrusted if not hostile.

The solution is to create some kind of barrier or *firewall* through which all connections to a network must pass. A firewall aims to stop the 'flames' from the untrusted network crossing over into the trusted network. Naturally, it will only work if absolutely all the communication between the two networks passes through the firewall. There are various types of firewall, ranging from a simple packet filtering firewall, which checks whether the data that is passing through comes from an acceptable address, to screened subnets, also known as DeMilitarised Zones (DMZs), consisting of an area protected by two simple firewalls. One routes traffic to and from the trusted network to a firewall in the screened subnet and another does the same for the traffic from the untrusted network. These are the kinds of firewall configuration that you would expect to find protecting a hospital network.

Protecting users: email attacks

Opening unknown attachments, often disguised as interesting pictures or documents, has been the main cause of very expensive security breaches resulting in worldwide networks being unavailable or slow to use. Common methods used to breach security include:

- *Viruses*: small computer program snippets that are designed to do some harm on their host system. They are usually attached to or hidden in ordinary files.
- *Trojan horses*: codes hidden in other useful programs, which have a destructive function of some sort.
- *Worms*: unlike viruses, these exist as separate entities and do not attach themselves to other files or programs. A worm can spread itself automatically over the

network from one computer to the next. Worms take advantage of automatic file sending and receiving features found on many computers, including email services.

Protecting users: Internet attacks

Although email is the usual culprit, malicious code can be imported from other applications, especially from web pages. Often this code takes the form of a program that will run in the background on host computers, collecting each keystroke entered and then sending these on to the attacker. These 'phishing' programs or 'spyware' are of great concern as they can capture user authentication details as well as confidential data. The best protection against these threats is provided by intrusion detection systems (IDS). Host-based intrusion detection systems check for the arrival of viruses, worms, and spyware as well as attempts to modify operating system software. Network intrusion detection systems are placed where they can take a copy of all the network traffic and look for patterns of activity known to signify an attack and also for unusual activity.

There are two main problems with intrusion detection systems. One is the maintenance cost of keeping the file of patterns up to date. The other is working out how to stop the system from signalling attacks that are not attacks, or missing the real attacks. Adjusting the *threshold* that balances the system between these two undesired behaviours can be tricky and will depend on the security goals to be achieved.

The informed consumer

From patient to consumer

A popular image of the ideal patient–doctor relationship sees the knowledgeable and caring physician counselling and guiding the trusting, compliant, and grateful patient.

Not any more! The patient of today comes to the health professional fresh from the Internet and armed not only with information about his or her condition, but also with information about the credentials of the health professional and possibly even with advice or a diagnosis already provided through an online consultation.

These developments are facilitating a change in the traditional relationship to one of mutual participation or even, with more assertive and knowledge-rich patients, to a relationship where the health professional becomes the adviser and the patient drives the relationship. This is indicated by the increasing use of the word *consumer* instead of the word *patient*.

Don't fight

The emergence of the consumer is an aspect of e-health that the health care system must respond to, rather than manage. So too are the information and commercial services that consumers are accessing. Health services and health professionals can respond in several ways. First, they can play ostriches and pretend that this aspect of e-health is not happening. Second, they can become defensive, perhaps hostile, and negate the information acquired by the consumer. Third, they can adopt a more positive role and assist the consumer to access reliable material and use it wisely.

Facilitate

There are two types of websites being accessed by consumers: commercial sites seeking to promote a health-related product or service, and information or education sites. There is sufficient overlap so that it can be extremely difficult for consumers to separate the pearls of wisdom from information that has a vested interest or bias.

There are even sites that begin offering high quality, unbiased information, but which, as a result of their popularity, succumb to offers of commercial sponsorship, which result in some questioning of their ongoing neutrality. An example is the site operated by the former US Surgeon General, Dr Koop. He initially set up the site to ensure a balanced view of the ever-growing field of medical information in the USA. Today he and his site are targets for serious accusations of commercial bias. It therefore becomes an issue for consumers to identify sites that offer reliable and unbiased education as against promotion of specific products or services. The health professional and the health care system can assist with this by sponsoring sites such as **MedlinePlus**, Healthfinder, and HealthInsite, which offer high quality information. They can also assist consumers to develop skills to evaluate websites themselves.

SUMMARY

E-health is capturing the imagination of government, health care services, health professionals, and consumers. Often it is the technology that is generating this interest. It is important when discussing e-health to remain focused on the problems and issues to be resolved.

E-health encompasses a wide range of activities and services, ranging from teleconferencing and videoconferencing to use of the Internet. Activities include clinical consultations, education, and information gathering. It includes services and activities conducted under the auspices of the established health care systems and those in the broader arena of commercial and business interests, community groups, and individuals. These individuals and groups use the Internet to offer activities, information, and services much wider in scope, much less coordinated, and much less controlled than those offered by traditional service systems.

There is limited evidence available to indicate the success of e-health. Existing evidence does suggest that applications and services are context specific, being more suited to some activities, professionals, and consumer groups in some situations than others.

Nevertheless, e-health is continuing to attract interest. The major drivers are commercial, business, and community groups, including consumers. The changing demographics and demands on services are also driving e-health.

Many groups driving e-health are also key players. Key players have different views of potential benefits and issues of e-health and these different views may conflict with each other. Key players range from those who shape policy and make funding decisions at a strategic level, to those who ensure that a service will be successful by using it. They will therefore have different levels of power and influence in presenting their views. Consequently some key players may shape (albeit inadvertently) services in a way that significantly disadvantages other groups.

Effective planning for an e-health service or application will involve key players, thus helping to ensure that different perspectives are considered. Planning will also enable a problem-solving focus rather than a technology focus by linking the proposed program to the strategic directions, outputs, and outcomes of the organisation, and using regular review and evaluation to keep the project on track.

As with any health care activity involving personal information, security must be a key focus for e-health. In addition to the issues around privacy and confidentiality, specific security issues for e-health relate to protecting networks and individual users from viruses and other attacks. Firewalls and intrusion detection systems are examples of techniques used.

Finally, e-health has seen the patient transform into the consumer. The emergence of the consumer is an aspect of e-health that the health care system must respond to, rather than manage. Health professionals can respond in several ways. They can ignore, resist, or actively encourage consumers in their quest for relevant and reliable information.

WWW LINKS

E-health, telehealth

Health Communication Network, Australia <http://www.hcn.net.au/>

John Mitchell and Associates, recent publications: E-Health <http://www.jma.com.au/ehealth_pubs.htm>

Roger Clarke's Home Page <http://www.anu.edu.au/people/Roger.Clarke/>

Telemedicine: creating virtual certainty out of remote possibilities <http://www.dhs.vic.gov.au/ahs/archive/telemed/execsum.htm>

Telemedicine Information Exchange <http://tie.telemed.org/>

Legal aspects

General Practice Computing Group, Australia, 'Legal issues in general practice computerisation' <http://www.gpcg.org/publications/docs/projects2001/GPCG_Project22_01_discussion_paper.pdf>

Standards

HL7 Australia <http://www.hl7.org.au/>

Canadian Institute for Health Information <http://secure.cihi.ca/cihiweb/>

New Zealand Health Information Service <http://www.nzhis.govt.nz/documentation/index.html>

HL7 United Kingdom <http://www.hl7.org.uk/>

HL7 USA <http://www.hl7.org/

American National Standards Institute (ANSI) <http://webstore.ansi.org/ansidocstore/dept.asp?dept_id=3104>

CRITICAL THINKING

Choose an e-health project that could be implemented in your local area.

1 What national and local drivers might influence the development of the project?

2 Who might be the key stakeholders? List benefits and drawbacks of the project from the perspective of each stakeholder group.

3 Identify any potential conflicts between various stakeholder perspectives. Consider how potential conflicts might be managed.

4 Draw up a project definition using the steps outlined in this chapter.

5 Develop a plan for implementation of the project, using the steps outlined in this chapter. Include strategies for evaluating the project.

CHAPTER 8

ELECTRONIC HEALTH RECORDS

OVERVIEW

The electronic health record (EHR) is arguably one of the most significant advances in medicine in the last decade. It is inevitable that in the very near future, most health providers around the world will have some form of electronic system for the collection, storage, and sharing of patient information. While there is broad agreement that an EHR is the way to go, there are many issues that must be resolved before such a record is successfully implemented. This chapter critically explores current issues relating to the development of an EHR.

OBJECTIVES

At the completion of this chapter, you should be able to:
- identify issues around the multiple use of paper-based records systems
- discuss types of electronic records in terms of their purpose, and levels of integration, automation, and connectivity
- differentiate between electronic records and electronic record summaries
- discuss issues to be considered when planning an electronic health record system
- discuss security issues specific to an electronic heath record
- describe issues around clinician adoption of an electronic health record.

CONCEPTS

Electronic health record
Centralised EHR
Electronic medical record
Distributed EHR
Electronic patient record

Patient-held smart card
Computer-based health record
Centralised EHR model
Distributed EHR model

INTRODUCTION

As with most other aspects of health informatics, the electronic health record is an evolving, multi-faceted, complex phenomenon. There are different views about what such a record is and how it should be used, and different organisations and facilities may seek different types of record. This will be so even if we succeed in developing and implementing the ultimate vision of:

> An electronic longitudinal collection of personal health information usually based on the individual, entered or accepted by health care providers, which can be distributed over a number of sites or aggregated at a particular source. The information is organised primarily to support continuing, efficient and quality health care. The record is under the control of the consumer and is stored and transmitted securely (National EHR Taskforce 2000, p. 21).

This chapter explores the evolving, multi-faceted, complex phenomenon of the EHR. In doing so, it considers the expectations and concerns of key players and discusses issues around the development and implementation of an electronic record. Many of the issues will apply to all but the most basic of computerised patient records, but will increase in complexity as the electronic record becomes increasingly integrated and more widely accessible.

The Australian government Health*Connect* website, Health Canada, and the United Kingdom NHS website (see WWW links at the end of the Chapter) have extensive documentation addressing many of the issues raised in this chapter. You are advised to access these sites.

USING ELECTRONIC RECORDS

This section begins by exploring the need for an EHR in the context of modern-day health care. It considers different ideas about what such a record is, and explores the current use of electronic records in the health care environment.

The 'holy grail'?

The EHR is coming. It is discussed as a *fait accompli*. Box 8.1 and Table 8.1 demonstrate the general belief that the EHR is the best thing since penicillin and we should all be jumping on the bandwagon.

There is need for reflection, however. The development and implementation of electronic health records involves dealing with many issues and challenges. First, it is necessary to determine why we need one. Then it is important to clarify exactly what is meant by an electronic health record and, by extension, what goes in one, where it is kept and who has access to it. In resolving these questions, issues of standards, privacy, and security will need to be addressed. The answers to many of these will vary depending on the health system you are talking about. The five health systems referred to

GOVERNMENTS

Australia

One of the key recommendations in Health*Online* is the development of a national framework for the use of electronic health records. Increasingly, the ability of electronic health records to improve the efficiency, safety and quality of care compared with paper-based systems is being recognised across the health sector (National Electronic Health Records Taskforce 2000, p. C4).

Canada

The Advisory Council on Health Infostructure identified the electronic health record to be of pivotal importance to an integrated health care delivery system. It is the means by which patient-centred health care delivery can be achieved. As such, the EHR is a priority for Health Canada as a key element of a Canadian health infostructure (Advisory Council on Health Infostructure 2001, p. 1).

New Zealand

As a result of New Zealand's new focus on seamless delivery of health care between primary and secondary providers, and increasing pressure for individuals to take responsibility for their own health status, both clinicians and consumers need access to up-to-date patient information and the latest health research. New Zealand EHRs are becoming increasingly technologically advanced (Kerr 2004).

United Kingdom

By 2010, every NHS patient in England will have an individual electronic NHS Care Record, announced Health Secretary John Reid today. This is a key part of reform of the NHS and will help make the NHS a truly responsive service that provides patients with more choice (UK Department of Health News 2003).

USA

Three months ago, President Bush set the goal for every American to have an electronic medical record—instead of a paper one—within ten years. To get there, the government will consider ways to encourage doctors and hospitals to make the investment in technology (Schmit & Appleby 2004).

Table 8.1 The health administrators

Priority	Australia (%)	Canada (%)	New Zealand (%)	United Kingdom (%)	USA (%)
Electronic medical records/IT	35	47	46	38	62
Emergency room/ operating room/ critical care facility	26	18	4	22	13
Basic hospital/ patient facilities	17	14	21	22	3
Diagnostic equipment/ medical technology	9	16	11	10	3

Source: Schoen et al. 2003, *Commonwealth Fund International Survey of Health Executives,* used with permission.

throughout this book will have different ideas, issues, and answers because they are structured and funded differently. Finally, the views of key stakeholders come into play. While governments and administrators are enthusiastic, other groups may have some reservations. Consider Roger Clarke's argument:

> On balance, it is likely that patients have something to gain from EHRs; but not as much as might be suggested by the technologies' proponents. What's more, consultations across a range of health consumer groups indicate that there is interest in these technologies being used to make emergency data more readily available, and to enable access to medication information and the results of diagnostic tests; but that scepticism exists about their use for detailed event summaries, let alone full health care records. Third parties, on the other hand, have a great deal to gain from the consolidation of patient data (2001, p. 2).

Why do we need one?

> Electronic Health Records (EHRs) are not an end in themselves but are a means of greatly enhancing many of the attributes we ascribe or aspire to in the traditional paper-based health record. These attributes include the support of communication between health care professionals, provision of a legal account of patient care, clinical decision support, enhanced efficiency of health care professionals, and support of health education, audit, and clinical research. All of this with the goal of improving the quality of patient care (Schloeffel 1998, p. 1).

Most of the shortcomings of paper-based records are now quite obvious, particularly to those still working with them. They include:

- *Duplication*: Each time an individual visits a new health professional or service, data, particularly identifying data, is recorded. This is time consuming for both the person collecting the data and the consumer.

- *Missing data*: Different people use different parts of the record. They may remove the sections they want. These might not be replaced for some time. They may even be lost.
- *Currency of information*: Data transfer is not always efficient. Someone might forget to post, fax, or electronically transfer the data; someone might leave it in the in-tray or filing tray until they get around to filing it; the health professional might have the file on his or her desk, so the new data cannot be filed.
- *Errors in data transfer*: Content errors are one form. Errors also occur if information is sent to the wrong file. The pathology lab might have two patients named Roberta. If someone is careless (or tired, or distracted), the test results might be mixed up. Illegible handwriting may also result in error.
- *Format for data presentation*: The lack of accepted standards or conventions means that data and information may well be recorded according to personal preferences. This may be very useful for the creator but not at all useful for anyone it is forwarded to.
- *Availability, accessibility*: Many different people use individual records. If one person is recording or reviewing content, no one else has access to it.
- *Security and confidentiality*: The loose pages and unduplicated contents of the paper-based record make it vulnerable. Records may be kept in a secure location but it can be difficult to monitor access. Patients' notes may be removed, handled, processed, and eventually re-filed by staff not involved with the care of that individual. When data needs to be communicated between facilities, it becomes even more vulnerable. It may sit in an in-tray or fax machine where anyone wandering past may pick it up and read it: 'Oh look! According to this fax, your neighbour has an STD!'.
- *Availability and access for secondary use*: Collecting, depersonalising, and aggregating data for secondary uses such as research and policy development is difficult and time consuming.

Many are viewing the electronic health record as the answer to these problems. Yet while the idea may appear straightforward, there are many issues to be resolved before the electronic record comes near to living up to the expectations held for it, not the least of which is deciding just what the term 'electronic health record' means.

What are we talking about?

> Who cares? I don't care what you want to call them. That's not my mission or my fight. I call them computer notes, but whatever you want to call them is fine by me (Naegele, in Marietti 1998, p. 1).

A vision or visions

Ask five people what they think an EHR is, and you may get five different answers, and quite possibly the answers will use five different terms. The EHR is an evolving entity. The first computerised patient records were simply electronic versions of the paper record and were created by entering data from paper documents. Today, efforts are being directed towards creating electronic records that contain a comprehensive collection of an individual's health information stored in a variety of formats, maintained by, and accessible to, multiple health professionals, and the consumer.

Table 8.2 Levels of integration, automation, and connectivity

Level	Characteristics
Automated medical record	Data is entered into a stand-alone computer from paper documents. The original documents and images are still stored and communicated using paper. This type of record does not alter the paper-based system used by the organisation.
Computerised patient record (CPR)	Paper documents are scanned into a computer. They can be accessed by more than one person at a time in different locations within a facility. This level of record offers quicker and more efficient retrieval of records without changing the basic structure of the paper-based system.
Electronic medical record (EMR)	Data is entered directly into the computer, and X-ray, pathology and pharmacy data can be integrated into the record. There may be paper back up. There is increased access within the facility and between facilities. More advanced records may incorporate functions such as clinical decision support, results reporting, and appointment scheduling.
Electronic patient record (EPR)	The level of integration enables all clinical data to be entered and stored electronically. The level of automation enables this record to operate across local/state/national/international boundaries. This level of record requires technologies for information data interchange.
Electronic health record (EHR)	This level of record represents a comprehensive, longitudinal collection of an individual's health information, including both medical and non-traditional health- and lifestyle-related information, with the consumer as the focus around which the information is recorded. The level of integration would enable data to be entered, accepted, and viewed by health care providers. Data and information might be distributed over a number of sites or aggregated at a particular source. The EHR supports a holistic approach to health care.

Source: adapted from Lewis & Mitchell 1998

One way of distinguishing between the types of records and the terms is to think of them as indicating different degrees of integration, automation, and connectivity. Levels of integration refer to:

- *Degree of integration of content*: Content integration can range from an automated record that acts as a replacement for an existing paper-based record (which may be able to be better organised and retrieved; may not include multi-media data; may not include data from other clinicians, unless scanned in), to an EHR, which includes the total health information for an individual (including multi-media files) that could be made available in the support of clinical activities.

- *Degree of integration of access*: Integration access can range from an automated file only available on an individual computer, through to records integrated across a facility, such as a general practice or an enterprise such as a hospital, to a fully-fledged national electronic record.

The degree of integration is dependent on the perceived purpose of the record, and the level of automation and connectivity that technology is able to provide. Table 8.2 suggests a schema for five levels of integration and automation while Box 8.2 describes two systems illustrating different levels of content and access integration.

BOX 8.2

DIFFERENT LEVELS OF CONTENT AND ACCESS INTEGRATION

Home telecare system

The home telecare system (HTS), developed at the University of New South Wales, integrates a range of e-health services and advanced information and communications technologies relevant to the management of chronic disease at home. Clinical measurements data as well as health status questionnaires and daily logs are scheduled remotely by the care team and, when completed in the patient's own home, are automatically synchronised and replicated at a secure central server over a standard telephone line. Data is processed, analysed, and added to a longitudinal health record. Authorised members of the care team can then review the data at any time from anywhere using a simple computer browser (Celler & Lovell 2003).

The Mosoriot Medical Record System, Eldoret, Kenya: capturing data to improve quality of care in sub-Saharan Africa

The Mosoriot Medical Record System (MMRS) is a computer-based patient record system within a primary care health centre in rural Kenya. The record has a modular structure, programmed in Microsoft Access. The modules include Patient Registration, Encounter (visit) Data, Reports and a core Data Dictionary. Each patient has a unique computer-generated MMRS number that provides identification in association with their personal details. The computer prints an identifying label with the unique number, which is affixed to the patient's MMRS identity tag. Patient encounters are intended to follow a strict sequential flow from registration desk to scheduled appointment, pharmacy, and final check-out through the financial window. Completed encounter forms are collected, relevant data is entered into the computer, and the encounter forms are returned to the patient (Hannan et al. 2002).

In the real world

Summer vacation season is approaching, and Americans soon will be hitting the road by the millions. As their vehicles cruise the open road a ritual will play out when some impatient young adventurer utters the illogical question, 'Are we there yet?' That is followed just as inevitably by, 'When are we gonna be there?' The same questions apply in health care to the subject of implementing computer-based patient records systems. The answer to the first question by all accounts is 'No,' we aren't there yet. The answer to the second, more pressing query is 'Get comfortable,' many experts say, because the destination might be as far away as the horizon (Briggs 2002, p. 56).

The answer to the question 'where are we?' probably depends on who you ask.

Today, most health care organisations and facilities, even quite small ones, have at least a basic level of computerised patient records. The focus of much current work is on expanding these into an electronic medical record and perhaps an electronic patient record. Issues revolve around the integration of disparate hardware and software, standards to enable the exchange of data, and security of information stored in records. Different versions of electronic records are currently being trialled or adopted in health systems around the world. Box 8.3 lists three of these.

BOX 8.3

EHR ACTIVITY

- The Children's Hospital at Westmead is expanding its electronic patient record to include paperless medical records. The new system captures the paper patient record as electronic images and makes this available instantly across the hospital and remotely (Children's Hospital at Westmead 2003).
- The Alberta Electronic Health Record is a province-wide clinical health information system that links physicians, pharmacists, hospitals, home care and other providers across the province. The record stores pertinent information online so that health care providers may access a patient's prescription history, allergies and laboratory test results immediately online, via computer (Alberta Government 2003).
- The New South Wales Department of Health will begin prototyping its new electronic health records project this month. The New South Wales implementation differs slightly from the national architecture. The online record is described as summary level, not a full record, and users are capable of defining who can see the information (Gedda 2004).

The influence of different national health structures is seen in Box 8.3. In Australia, the joint state–federal responsibilities for health are seeing EHR trials at both levels, and not always in coordination with one another. This will create unique problems for the Australian system.

In addition, many national governments, as seen in Box 8.1, are advocating and planning for the broader vision of an electronic patient record or an electronic health record. There is strong support for the concept. However, there are also concerns and issues, with some suggesting that the concept of a national integrated health record is unrealistic. The issues still to be addressed range from technical aspects to questions about the accuracy of the espoused benefits and who are the real beneficiaries of an electronic health record.

Another dimension: replacements and summaries

While the various types of electronic health records are often presented as a continuum, there are in fact two types of systems being discussed. One is the replacement of the paper used in the day-to-day management of patient care with electronic equivalents. This is relatively straightforward in specific areas where there is already an electronic component to what is being done. In pathology disciplines, such as clinical chemistry and haematology, patient results are largely generated as digital information by computerised analysers. The step from paper-result delivery to electronic is minimal. Similarly, in the management of radiotherapy, computerised planning of patient treatment is the norm, and electronic management of all aspects of the process of treating patients is a relatively small step. However, in a hospital ward, most of the work of looking after a patient is still driven by paper forms. Nursing and medical record keeping is still largely a process that uses paper. For some time to come, the health record in this context will include a paper component.

The second type of EHR is the summary of a patient's health events and outcomes over time. This is often the model envisaged for national electronic health record systems. Creating an electronic summary at the end of an interaction with a patient is no great burden if it is a 15-minute activity at the end of a hospital stay of several days. Usually, all of the information about the patient's treatment will be together in one paper (or electronic) file. However, if the patient encounter is a standard GP consultation (which many GPs view as barely long enough to effectively manage their patients' problems) then additional time spent creating an electronic summary of the encounter with each patient will not be a welcome addition to the work day. The key to success in this setting will be to integrate a form of electronic record-keeping into the workflow in a way that does not interfere with communication between clinician and patient, and does not appreciably add to the cost of delivering the service (or the time taken).

There are widely differing views on the possibility and viability of a fully-fledged EHR. Views range from the optimistic expectation of national electronic records in many countries within the next few years, to the view that this is an impossible dream and that efforts are more appropriately focused on lesser levels of integration and connectivity.

IDENTIFYING PARAMETERS

> The different health care constituents value CPR components differently. While the physician group practice of fewer than ten physicians may be able to achieve a paperless environment with a simple EMR system, the emerging IDN has higher expectations of the CPR. Enterprise capability requires that hundreds of physicians and nurses participate in the roll-out in order to string together the disparate organisational departments (Gaillour 1999, p. 23).

This section focuses on the issues and processes around establishing the parameters of an EHR. These may vary in relevance and complexity, depending on the level of record being considered and the organisational context in which it is being developed, yet most are relevant to all but the most basic level of automated record. The emphasis is on the use of effective planning to identify and seek to resolve issues, particularly those arising from various key player perspectives.

Planning

Planning is good. It clarifies what is going to be done, by whom, and with what outcomes. One approach to planning for an electronic health record is to focus on technical issues such as:

- agreeing about data to be gathered
- adopting relevant data standards
- developing standard architectures
- networking
- storage
- privacy and confidentiality.

In Australia, the National Electronic Health Records Task Force produced an issues paper, 'A Health Information network for Australia', which discusses these issues in Appendix 3 (2000). It is a document well worth reading (see the WWW links at the end of the chapter).

These technology issues can also be addressed by adopting a problem driven approach. From this perspective, the initial phases of planning will begin with questions such as:

- What is the record expected to do?
- What goes into it?
- Who will use it?
- What security and other standards are needed?

It is somewhat artificial to consider these questions individually. What goes into a record will be influenced by the purpose of the record, the level of integration and information-sharing required, the model selected for the record, and decisions around access and control. On the other hand, the questions provide a framework for the systematic discussion of issues and ensure a problem-solving focus rather than a technology-oriented one.

What is the record expected to do?

The scale and context of a health care facility will shape the requirements of the EHR. Factors to be considered include the location, size, and purpose of the facility, existing levels of automation, access requirements, and available technology. Facilities may range from a single rural general practice to large metropolitan hospitals to specialist practices such as pathology and radiography services. They will have varying levels of automation, with some environments still largely paper driven, while others generate most, if not all, information digitally. Some facilities will have access to sophisticated hardware, software, and networks capable of transmitting large amounts of data, while others will have much more limited capabilities. Access requirements may range from a single user to multiple users distributed across a large facility.

Some systems are intended to replace the existing paper systems used in the day-to-day management of patients within the facility. Others will be perceived as forming the basis of a patient record with much broader application and access, and consist of a summary of a patient's health events and outcomes over time.

Decisions about what the record is expected to do will shape answers to questions of content, control, and access. Box 8.4 represents one view.

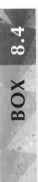

BOX 8.4

WHAT SHOULD AN EHR DO?

There is clear support for Health*Connect* operating as a passive store rather than actively interpreting clinical information or initiating transfers of EHR information from provider systems. There is clear support for Health*Connect* being kept as simple as possible and not attempting to deliver optional functions such as clinical decision support. Provider systems should deliver optional support functions. Health*Connect* needed to provide EHR information to support these functions (Health*Connect*, 2004).

What goes into the record?

The question of what goes into a record will depend on the perceived purpose of the record and the degree of integration of its contents. With less integrated records, the issue of content may be less of a problem, since access would be limited to individual facilities or at most a few facilities. The option of more integrated records, allowing access to greater numbers of health professionals at a wider range of locations, does raise some issues. The purpose of storing information is to assist with decisions about future care, and the focus should be on collecting personal health information that both consumers and health care providers consider to be necessary and useful. This raises the question of what is necessary and useful. In response to this question, some might answer 'Why, everything, of course'. Others will not be so sure.

For many health professionals it is important to have as much information about the patient as possible, especially as material that may appear insignificant or irrelevant to the patient may sometimes be vital for the diagnosis of a problem. Box 8.5 illustrates this.

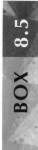

HOW MUCH INFORMATION?

Consider the situation of a patient who appears disoriented, confused or, worse still, unconscious, who has in fact been treated elsewhere for drug addiction and there is no mention of this in the patient's record at the location where they present. Of course, this does happen all of the time, and most health professionals are skilled in sorting out these kinds of issues, but it may take up vital time, often unnecessary laboratory testing, and possibly risks to the outcome for that patient.

Yet there are concerns about certain data and information being included when a number of individuals are able to access the material. Electronic records systems manage the type of data that has been used to discriminate against people. Unfortunately it is not easy to determine which types of data, if accessed without authorisation, could cause some kind of harm. Everyone has a particular set of circumstances that determine what may or may not be considered sensitive information. Even apparently innocuous data can do harm.

There are two types of data that may be stored in an electronic record. These are non-health data and health data and information.

Non-health data

Non-health data is basic data said to be necessary if the record is to be workable. This includes time, date, ID of provider and consumer, location of health service, any coding system used, and access authority. Yet this seemingly innocuous information can be contentious:

> The fact that a person was treated in a particular hospital or location, such as a prison or sexual health centre, could indirectly reveal information about the person. Therefore, even though summary information such as name of hospital and health provider may not appear to be 'health information' as such, to the extent that it reveals something about a person's health status it may need to be treated with the same sensitivity as other health information (NSW Ministerial Advisory Committee 2000, p. 11).

Health data and information

There is a broad range of data that constitutes 'health information'. This might include details not only of medical diagnoses and treatment but also social and lifestyle factors, including information about domestic violence, drug use, cultural and religious beliefs, and socio-economic factors. The health professional perspective may consider this to be essential information. The health consumer may not.

Excluded data

It can be assumed that not all data related to a consumer will be included in the electronic record. There are two possibilities for data that is not to be included. The first is that it is destroyed. This may indeed be appropriate in some cases. However, there will also be data that, while it is considered too sensitive to include on an electronic medical record, is nevertheless essential for the well-being of the consumer and should therefore be recorded in relevant locations. Box 8.6 illustrates this.

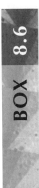

BOX 8.6

SENSITIVE INFORMATION

There still is a need for the clinician to write information such as a possible concern that a child may be the victim of abuse, so that he or she and others will be alerted to that possibility should the child return with 'suspicious' symptoms and signs. Imagine if the parent (especially if he or she were the abuser) were to have access to this kind of information. Even worse, imagine if the parent had access and did not know about the suspicion of abuse. What if there was in fact no abuse at all!

This suggests that health enterprises and health professionals will need to continue to maintain medical records outside the boundary of the electronic record. A record that utilises summaries of a patient's health events and outcomes over time, with comprehensive records kept by individual health providers, would enable sensitive information to be quarantined. It would also create the possibility that not all relevant information is available to the health professional. Important information contained in the health provider notes may not be in the summaries.

In a longitudinal record, the question of currency of information may also become an issue. Essential information at one point (a viral upper respiratory infection as a child, for example) may be less relevant as time goes by. Retaining all possible information in a longitudinal record may make little sense. There is also a danger here. Health data that we are happy to share now may become a liability in the future. An example of this is the use, by Western Australian police, of heel prick samples taken from all newborn babies (Guthrie tests) and stored for decades as personally identified data. This material was recently used to match DNA samples taken from a crime scene (Phillips 2003, p. 1).

Ownership, control, and access

The ownership of electronic health records is a complex issue, since electronic data can be copied very simply and the copy is indistinguishable from the original (National Electronic Health Records Taskforce 2000, p. 75).

Until recently there was no issue about ownership of medical records. The person who created it, usually the health practitioner, owned it. With an electronic record, there is a view that the patient will be the owner. Yet in the evolving electronic environment, with increased information sharing and ability to duplicate information, ownership may no longer be relevant. Control and access may be more useful concepts.

Until the electronic health record began to evolve, it was assumed that, as with ownership, the individual or organisation creating the record controlled what went into it, and who was able to view the contents. There was therefore relatively little concern about what was written in records and how it was recorded, and the notes were often very 'personal', not meant to be seen by anyone else.

An underlying theme of the discussion around EHRs is that people should have access to their own information and must be able to control who can see it. This gives rise to several issues. First, depending on the model of record adopted, some health professionals may feel it necessary to modify the contents of medical records to accommodate consumer access. It will be necessary to be more careful about what is written and how it is written. This may not be a bad thing. However, as Box 8.7 shows, it may have an unforseen influence on communication between health professionals.

BOX 8.7

ACCESS

When a patient initiates a consultation with a physician the diagnosis may not be immediately obvious, so after taking a thorough history and completing a physical examination, the physician will reach a differential diagnosis, which will be further refined by the results of some tests. The contents of the differential diagnosis will usually include the actual cause of the patient's complaint, but there will be other conditions in the list as well. The physician may want to exclude serious and dangerous conditions before telling his patient that he believes the condition to be something ordinary and easily cured. If the patient has full access to his or her record, he or she could be seriously and unnecessarily stressed to discover that the physician is even considering, for example, cancer. The differential diagnosis is an important part of a medical record as it not only assists the physician involved in recalling details of the patient, but other clinicians find it useful to know what their colleague was considering at the time, should they become involved with the patient subsequently.

A second issue relates to consumer consent over access to the record. Consumer consent and control over access to the electronic record is a key element of most national initiatives, as shown in Box 8.8.

CONSENT AND CONTROL OF ACCESS

Australia

In the context of Health*Connect*, consent involves health care providers seeking the agreement of consumers to record their information on the Health*Connect* network and to access that information from the network in the future. Consent must be informed and voluntary, with participation in Health*Connect* for both consumers and providers to be on an 'opt-in' basis (Health*Connect* 2004).

Canada

Privacy is the most important policy area that needs to be addressed in relation to EHRs. Without public support on how privacy will be addressed, EHR systems will not be able to proceed. Privacy involves the right of individuals to determine when, how and to what extent they share information about themselves and others (Health Canada 2001).

New Zealand

The challenging elements of the [electronic health record] mainly involve security issues. There needs to be protection for all of those interacting with the record. The consumer, most of all, must know that their record is available only to authorised users, and that any publication, either paper or electronic, must be only with their informed consent (Gillies & Holt 2003)

The following are examples of situations where consent of the health consumer would be required:

- health professionals requesting access to a consumer's record
- health practitioners sharing health information with other health practitioners
- bringing together public health information (for example, births or cancer registry information) with information gathered from individual health encounters
- health administrators, researchers, statisticians, and policy advisers 'mining' health data.

The requirement for consent will ensure that the consumer feels confident that his or her information is not accessed inappropriately. Yet this same requirement has the potential to impact on quality of service, since consumers may deny access to specific information, due to concerns about confidentiality.

The type of record used will influence decisions about access. A more comprehensive and integrated record may generate questions such as 'Which health professionals?', 'Which information?', or 'Does your dentist need to know you had an abortion fifteen years ago?'

How will it work?

Models for an EHR are often discussed in terms of degree of centralisation or distribution.

The centralised EHR

As the name suggests, a centralised EHR sees comprehensive patient data collected and stored in a single repository or location. Individual service providers or health professionals maintain the full details of individual encounters in their own electronic patient records, which are essentially subsets of the EHR. Authorised individuals (health professionals and consumer) are able to access these subsets to view the more detailed information contained within them. Figure 8.1 depicts a centralised electronic health records model.

Figure 8.1 Centralised model

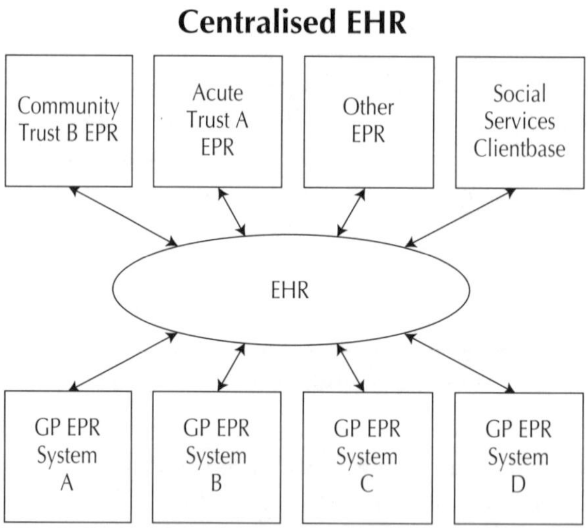

Centralised EHR

Source: from Protti 2002

Schloeffel suggests that few people would seriously advocate a fully centralised model where literally every clinical item for a lifetime is stored in a single data repository (1998, p. 4). Think about it!

The fully distributed EHR

In the distributed model, no location is considered to be the primary repository of information. Instead, the EHR is physically distributed across several sites. Users create their own view or record by accessing the data from these sites. Figure 8.2 depicts this model.

Figure 8.2 Distributed EHR

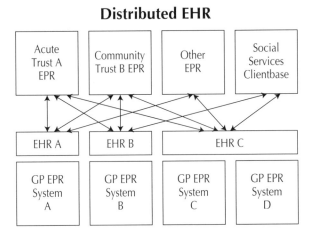

Source: from Protti 2002

Patient-held (smart) cards

Several European countries have been experimenting with the use of 'smart' card technology for several years. Kelly (2002, p. 64) identifies two main types of card. These are smart cards and magnetic strip cards. Magnetic strip cards can store only a limited amount of data. Smart cards contain a computer chip and are capable of storing significantly more data but can only be accessed using a card reader. Smart cards are said to offer benefits in terms of more effective patient identification, via basic administrative data stored on the card, instantly accessible vital data in the event of an emergency, and enhanced security. This latter point, however, is not necessarily supported by consumers: 'The idea of carrying around identifiable patient information raised the issue of civil liberties. Some respondents felt that they would not want to carry identifying information with them—people can steal your identity' (NHS National Programme for Information Technology 2003, p. 12).

The model adopted for the electronic health record will influence storage issues. A distributed system would see data stored at various locations and linked across a network when required. The New South Wales Ministerial Advisory Committee on Privacy and Health Information (2000, p. 9) suggests that this model minimises risks of breaches of privacy by allowing the consumer and health care provider to have more control over information transmitted to others. A centralised model would remove the control of information from the consumer, *increasing the risk of the information being inappropriately accessed by other parties* (2000, p. 9).

> The 2004/05 CIP work program includes the development of the clinical content of the shared EHR for Health*Connect* and jurisdictional information exchange. The shared EHR is not a comprehensive patient record, rather a summary of patient information derived from health care events relevant to ongoing care and captured in the form of 'health event summaries'. The collection of health event summaries relating to an individual will constitute their shared EHR (NSW Ministerial Advisory Committee on Privacy and Health Information 2000, p. 8).

This is an important issue. As the New South Wales Ministerial Advisory Committee on Privacy and Health Information (2000, p. 8) suggests, with the electronic format for health records, there may be increasing pressure and demands placed on the information by non-health care bodies (for example, insurers, employers, law enforcement agencies, and some government agencies).

Standards

> Data standards will be required in order to achieve any useful integration of data from different sources (Health*Connect* Taskforce 2000).

Electronic exchange of data requires standards. This is a complex challenge. Standards for paper-based records are basically spelling, grammar, and legibility (and not even that, if the record is for only one individual). Standards for electronic records include:

- clinical vocabularies
- structure and content standards
- messaging standards
- security standards.

This discussion focuses on structure and content standards, clinical vocabularies, and security issues specific to the electronic health record.

Structure and content

Structure and content standards were discussed in Chapter 6. With regard to the electronic health record, it should be noted that current efforts are focusing on developing interoperability at the level of *architectures*, rather than detailed data structures. An electronic record architecture, for example, is a model of the generic features necessary in a health record, but does not specify what must be stored in the record, or how a system should be implemented. The Good European Health Record (GEHR) is an example of architecture-driven electronic records using an object-oriented approach. Australia, Canada, New Zealand, and the USA have similar projects.

See the WWW links at the end of the chapter for more information.

Vocabularies

If information is to be useful and reliable, it must be accurately recorded and clearly understood. To do this, terms need to be used consistently. This is a problem for many clinicians, particularly those in specialised areas such as psychiatry, who frequently record their observations in narrative form, often using shorthand and their own particular jargon. For many, the ability to do so is considered an essential element for the successful practice of their discipline. However, narrative-style records may make it difficult to share data. There is no guarantee that others will interpret the free-form information in the same way. Standardisation of terminology is therefore seen to be an essential requirement for electronic records. This has seen efforts to develop a standardised universal vocabulary.

Today, there are more than 150 clinical vocabularies in use around the world. Many of these have been created for a specific purpose and contain levels of detail and nuances that reflect that purpose. Many of these vocabularies are used at national and international level, and their contents continue to expand.

Two examples of vocabularies used at an international level are Logical Observation Identifier Names and Codes (LOINC) and Systematised Nomenclature of Medicine (SNOMED).

LOINC is a standardised set of names and codes for laboratory tests and clinical observations, which was developed in mid-1995, while SNOMED is a reference medical terminology set developed more than twenty years ago and enhanced continually ever since. SNOMED is a formalised set of more than 300 000 coded medical terms, but is still found wanting by health care professionals who have specific requirements in order to carry out their work.

Given the number of clinical vocabularies, none of which adequately meet the needs of all health professionals, there is an increasing view that a universal vocabulary may be unrealistic. Coiera (2003, p. 217) also suggests that even if an acceptable universal vocabulary were to be defined then there is the problem of training all involved to use the standard terms consistently.

A possible solution is to abandon the idea of one standard health vocabulary and follow the idea of standards that match system purpose. After all:

> The essential goal is to have an acceptable code system for each kind of data. It is not necessary (it may not even be desirable) to have all of the codes come from a single master code system, because computers can integrate multiple code systems easily while avoiding collisions among assigned codes by adding a code source designation (American Nurses Association 1995).

Security

A universal electronic health record system relies upon security techniques to provide for the confidentiality of the data it records as it is stored and shared across networks; to authenticate users in an open system with an unknown number of authorised users;

and to provide for the integrity of the data on the records, and to ensure the availability of the records to authenticated users, in accordance with the provisions of privacy legislation. Cryptography plays a major role in helping to achieve these goals but can only do so once the process in which it is to be used has been defined. Many of the implementation problems with a universal electronic health record system lie in defining just what these processes should be.

The whole concept of electronic health records in any of their many varieties would be a great deal simpler if security issues could be either ignored or easily dealt with. Issues of privacy and confidentiality of information provide real challenges as each access to a record should only be made in the knowledge of patient consent to view. The trouble is that in practice an individual finds it hard to consider the implications of providing or denying consent as needs and circumstances change.

An interesting challenge is in providing for the integrity of the data on electronic health records. To be of use, clinicians are going to have to trust the data that they contain and make significant decisions on the basis of these data. Security techniques will be required to both provide for integrity of data and to indicate how incorrect data were recorded. Finally, the availability of the current record at the time and place of need is a problem that can be exacerbated by differing standards and formats as data travels across health authority boundaries.

Privacy and confidentiality

Deciding on what information should be kept confidential is not always straightforward. The confidentiality restrictions that people may want to place on access to their universal electronic health record can vary enormously and may not remain static over time. The privacy legislation acknowledges this by requiring health care practitioners to access PID only with the consent of the individual concerned.

In practice, however, there are difficulties in developing an effective and efficient method for obtaining patient consent. The model that requires patient consent for every single access of an electronic record is cumbersome and time consuming. On the other hand, a blanket consent model does not allow for changes in confidentiality requirements that may arise due to changed circumstances.

The technology to enable the kind of fine-grained control over the confidentiality of PID in health systems that some citizens require is not available. There have been some attempts to set up general purpose solutions for this that will sit between the applications using an electronic health record and the operating system. This is known as 'middleware'. These solutions use cryptography to provide for a user-controlled definition of consent to view each item of shared personally identified health data such as that used on a universal electronic health record.

Authentication

Passwords are the most common form of user verification. Yet passwords are vulnerable, since people often choose passwords that can easily be guessed, share passwords, write them down and leave them in visible places, use 'the remember this password' feature in applications, and cheerfully send them in plain text across unsecured networks.

A solution to the password problem is public key infrastructure (PKI), which allows users to be identified via a cryptographic key. Electronic health records can be protected by having users access the record using a secret key known only to them. The use of a private encoding is known as a signature. This is much harder to steal as it is generated and managed by software. In Australia, the Health Insurance Commission has contracted Health eSignature Authority (HeSA) and SecureNet to set up and support a PKI system that can effectively be used in health applications. See the WWW links at the end of the chapter for more detail on PKI.

Integrity

The concept of integrity of the data in an electronic health record is intriguing since much of the data is based on expert opinion. The opinion might be completely accurate when entered but become less so in the light of additional knowledge becoming available. The opinion might also be incorrect. Another example is measurements. These too may be suspect. The measurement might be recorded accurately but is of no use if the machine that produced it is wrongly calibrated. Security techniques cannot help with this aspect of data integrity. Their focus is on trying to ensure that data, once in a system, is not changed, created, or deleted in a fraudulent manner.

Availability

It is generally accepted that for maximum value, the EHR does need to be available to authorised users who may well be located at significant distances from the source of the data, thereby making it impractical to have a 'closed' system. A Virtual Private Network (VPN) is a reasonably practical option where a temporary single link is made between the user and the database. If that link is threatened, it immediately stops functioning, so the link is broken and the intruder, theoretically, cannot enter the system. A potential problem with this kind of link is that while the EHR may appear to be a single entity, in fact most likely it will be an aggregation of data that may well be stored in several places, and there could be issues of access control. For example, it is appropriate that radiological material (data) be stored in a specifically designed database, and similarly laboratory data has specific requirements. Access to the EHR gives the authorised user the ability to go to these other databases and see information that is stored there about the particular patient. It does not make sense to have this material stored in several places, or 'copied' somewhere.

STAKEHOLDER PERSPECTIVES

If EHRs have such an impressive list of benefits and capabilities, why has implementation of full-fledged systems been so slow? (Waegemann 2003, p. 2)

This final section considers the social and organisational aspects of introducing and operating an electronic health records system. As with other socio-technical systems in the health care environment, there are different perspectives that need to be accommodated. These include:

- patients/consumers
- health practitioners
- health administrator and managers
- national and state governments/health service providers.

Stakeholders share some issues, but have a different perspective on what the issue is and how it should be managed.

Patients/consumers

Electronic records are expected to result in improved quality of health care for consumers and a more consumer-focused health care system. Such a record may not, however, provide all the consumer benefits originally envisaged. Concerns include:

- There is no guarantee that all relevant information will be available to the health professional. In the proposed Australian model, for example, it is proposed that health summaries will form the electronic record. This creates the possibility of important information contained in the health provider notes not being available on summaries. In addition, consumers may deny access to specific information, or health care providers may withhold some information from the summaries due to concerns about confidentiality.
- Roger Clarke (2001) points to the possibility that in order to avoid information they consider sensitive going into an electronic record, consumers will put off seeking treatment. This could result in deterioration rather than an improvement in the quality of health care and, in the case of communicable diseases, pose public health issues.
- The consequences of breaches of privacy and confidentiality are significant for the consumer. These range from embarrassment arising from disclosure, even publication, of sensitive information, to serious discrimination, including bias by health carers, employees of welfare organisations, and employers. Enquiries have shown that abuse of personal health information is not uncommon, and offenders are often organisations (such as banks) that should know better.

Health professionals

> With my limited time, should I learn about a new medication which will immediately assist my 300 asthma patients, or learn the standards to enable me to record electronically that which I now do manually and which my office staff can then organise? (Waegemann 2003, p. 4)

Issues for health professionals include:

- *Lack of relevant information*: The other side of the coin is the possibility of a comprehensive history, particularly in the case of chronic conditions, resulting in the health professional being swamped with information. Health professionals are only human. In the busy clinical environment, faced with a mass of information, they may well tend to look for the most obvious and overlook some crucial smaller details.

- *Workflow and work routines*: While few health professionals would not welcome more effective and more efficient clinical procedures, the changes imposed by an electronic system may still provoke resistance. For example, clinicians may ask questions in a particular order and use their own individual terminology or short-hand for recording the answers. An electronic record may require questions to be asked in a different order, and to use standard terminology for recording responses.
- *Perceived value*: Moving from the traditional to the electronic version of the health record requires a very major change in one's work pattern, no matter how well this process is actually managed. If clinicians cannot see any personal reason for the change, and especially if they have not had any involvement in the decision to adopt an electronic record, they may well resist the process:

> There is currently great pressure on medical groups and health plans to invest in EMR systems. The administrative, scheduling, accounting and management advantages these systems offer are formidable. However, the EMR system installed in my office this year has very limited clinical decision support capability, and its potential use as a powerful tool for visit planning or active outreach to patients has yet to be operationalised. Will it make me a better doctor? So far, the answer is no (O'Connor 2003, p. 1).

Health administrators and managers

Issues for health administrators and managers include:

- *Security and confidentiality*: With the advent of increasingly integrated systems, and particularly the increasing trend to use the Internet to transmit information rapidly and widely, security is a significant issue for management.
- *Compatibility of systems*: Many health and medical organisations operate with a patchwork of legacy databases and systems that are often not compatible with one another. When moving towards more integrated data collection and information sharing, these legacy systems must be considered. Often they have been expensive to install, are still performing adequately, staff have become familiar with them, and they contain much valuable information. This becomes a particular problem for management where integration across services is contemplated.
- *Ownership and maintenance*: Management must deal with the issue of ownership and maintenance. The integrated electronic record will only be useful if it contains up-to-date relevant information. Patient ownership and/or control of their record may create difficulties for organisations. The issue of legal liability may be a mine-field in this environment.

At the beginning of this chapter, Roger Clarke's suggestion that health administration is the major beneficiary of electronic health records was introduced. Others agree.

In an interesting example of what George Orwell famously termed 'newspeak', proponents almost universally describe these proposals as facilitating an 'individual' or 'consumer' focus in health care. Yet the primary purpose of this new consumer focus is not necessarily benefit to the individual consumer at all (though this is often assumed to be an obvious ancillary benefit (Carter 2000, p. 28).

Carter refers to an early Health*Connect* project, which created electronic linkages between the Health Insurance Commission, medical practitioners, and pharmacists. The intention of this project was to minimise adverse events due to inappropriate prescribing. Carter observed, however, that the project's major activity had been electronic checking of consumer entitlements to medications at concession rates.

National and state governments/health service providers

Issues for national and state governments and health service providers relate to jurisdictional issues arising from the division of state and federal government responsibilities for funding and delivery of health services, and the existence of private and public systems that may be subject to different funding arrangements and regulations. Issues include overall responsibility for funding of infrastructure costs, establishment of appropriate standards to facilitate effective information exchange, and dealing with legal jurisdictions. As Bentivoglio observes, 'numerous studies have found that a complicated patchwork of State and federal laws and regulations is standing in the way of Internet-based health care. Many States still have so-called quill-and-pen laws that require various health care forms to be submitted on paper' (2003, p. 1).

SUMMARY

There is general agreement that a system serving multiple users of paper-based health records creates issues around availability, accessibility, incomplete or incorrect data, and duplication of data. The electronic record is being viewed as the answer to these issues.

An electronic health record can take many forms. One way of distinguishing between the types of records and the terms used is to think of them as indicating different degrees of integration, automation, and connectivity. The degree of integration is dependent on the perceived purpose of the record, and the level of automation and connectivity that available technology is able to provide.

While the various types of electronic health records are often presented as a continuum, there are two types of systems being discussed. One is the replacement of the paper used in the day-to-day management of patient care with electronic equivalents. The second type of EHR is the summary of a patient's health events and outcomes over time. This is often the model envisaged for national electronic health record systems.

Different health facilities will find that they require different types of record. This will be influenced by the intended purpose of the record, the level of integration and information-sharing required, the model selected for the record, and decisions around access and control.

Planning is the means for identifying these parameters and ensuring that they are met. Questions to be addressed when planning the record include issues about the data to be included, access and control issues, and technical issues around architecture, standards and security.

User buy-in is a significant factor in the successful implementation of an EHR. Users include consumers and health professionals and management. Consumers views need to be addressed, particularly in those systems that adopt an opt-in rather than an opt-out model. Health professionals will have issues around work processes and routines, but perhaps of more significance, around access to relevant and accurate data and information. Management face issues around ensuring both security and accessibility of information, resourcing appropriate technology, and managing issues around ownership and access.

WWW LINKS

National approaches

Health*Connect*, Australia <http://www.healthconnect.gov.au/pdf/ehr_rep.pdf>
Canada EHR: Electronic Health Record <http://www.infoway-inforoute.ca/ehr/index.php?lang=en>
New Zealand Health <http://www.moh.govt.nz/moh.nsf>
UK NHS Information Authority's Electronic Record Development and Implementation Programme
    <http://www.nhsia.nhs.uk/erdip/pages/default.asp>

Architecture

The Open EHR Community <http://www.openehr.org/index.html>

Issues

Carter, M. 2000, Integrated Electronic Health Records and Patient Privacy: Possible Benefits But Real Danger, MJA online <http://www.mja.com.au/public/issues/172_01_030100/carter/carter.html>
Clarke, R. 2001, 'Conventional public key infrastructure: an artefact ill-fitted to the needs of the information society' <http://www.anu.edu.au/people/Roger.Clarke/II/PKIMisFit.html>
Public Key Infrastructure (PKI) Security http://www.hic.gov.au/providers/online_initiatives/pki_security.htm>

CRITICAL THINKING

1 What are the advantages and disadvantages of a distributed system compared with a centralised system of electronic health records?

2 Will public key infrastructure (PKI) guarantee the security of health data stored in an electronic health record? Why/why not?

3 How would you balance the right of the consumer to have control over data in his or her own health record with the requirements for adequate information to enable the clinician to provide safe and effective health care?

4 What type of electronic record would you, as a health consumer, feel comfortable with?

CHAPTER 9

DECISION SUPPORT SYSTEMS

OVERVIEW

The evolution of decision support systems (DSSs) reflects the evolution of the discipline of health informatics. As with health informatics generally, the development of decision support systems has emerged from a multi-disciplinary base, with the most influential disciplines being artificial intelligence (AI) and information systems. Again, as with the broader discipline of health informatics, much of the early work was influenced by a technological perspective. Over time, the influence of the discipline of information systems has contributed to a more socio-technical perspective. Many of the issues and challenges arising from the introduction of decision support systems, particularly clinical support systems, are those shared by the discipline of health informatics. Despite evidence to indicate their usefulness, decision support systems, as with so many information management applications, have been slow to integrate into the mainstream clinical environment.

The development of decision support systems is a specialised field, requiring specific technical skills and knowledge. This chapter is a general overview of that field as it applies to health informatics. There are many specific references for those seeking a detailed analysis of the techniques and technologies of decision support systems. Several are included in the text and in the WWW links at the end of the chapter.

OBJECTIVES

At the completion of this chapter, you should be able to understand:
- the potential role of decision support systems in the administrative and clinical health environment
- current trends in the use of artificial intelligence and decision support systems in health care
- basic components of a decision support system
- the functionality and effectiveness of decision support systems in a clinical setting
- issues relating to the use of expert systems and decision support systems in the health environment.

CONCEPTS

Decisions support system   Fuzzy logic
Neural network   Artificial intelligence
Expert system   Intelligent agent

INTRODUCTION

This chapter explores the use of decision support systems in the health care environment. While the discussion identifies a range of applications, the emphasis is on clinical decision support. The first part of the chapter seeks to establish a context for the discussion by exploring perspectives and definitions of decision support systems. The discussion then focuses on the application of decision support systems in the health care environment, particularly the clinical environment. The final section discusses issues arising from the use of decision support systems in the clinical environment.

ABOUT DECISION SUPPORT SYSTEMS

As with many aspects of health informatics, the field of decision support systems has a multi-disciplinary base. In particular, the disciplines of artificial intelligence (AI) and information systems have shaped the development of decision support systems.

Artificial intelligence and decision support

In Chapters 2 and 3, the relationship between knowledge, information, and data was discussed. It was noted that data is combined to produce information while analysis and interpretation of information produces knowledge. It has been widely assumed that human intelligence is required to bring this understanding to information: 'When a health professional is given the information, understands the implications and possible outcome of the temperature pattern, and initiates an intervention for an elevated temperature, we have an example of medical domain knowledge' (Watson 2002, p. 26).

The field of artificial intelligence premises that it is possible to create machines that can simulate human intelligence. Therefore, artificial intelligence is concerned with the study of intelligent behaviour and knowledge engineering to develop knowledge-based systems. There are two branches of AI. Weak AI takes the view that some thinking-like functions can be programmed into computers, while strong AI believes that computers can be made to think on a level (at least) equal to humans. Early work in **clinical decision support systems** (CDSSs) was very much influenced by strong AI, and there were expectations that decision support systems would eventually replace doctors—the doctor-in-a-box concept.

A wide spectrum of systems can be included under the heading of AI. These range from complex systems such as expert systems, neural networks, fuzzy logic, and case-based reasoning, to simple intelligent agents that seek patterns or specific data.

AI techniques are increasingly being used in clinical applications to improve health and medical care. A specific area of AI is artificial intelligence in medicine (AIM), which focuses on developing systems that can be used in the clinical environment. Box 9.1 describes two examples.

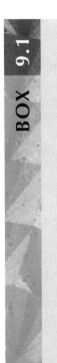

EXAMPLES OF DECISION SUPPORT SYSTEMS

Artificial intelligence methodologies were adopted to develop knowledge-based computer systems capable of interpreting medical images using representations of anatomical structures separate from image processing. This permits the same model to be used for several different imaging modalities, and results in a system that treats the analysis of images in a manner analogous to a human expert (Wilson 1999).

'Mentor' is a rudimentary decision support system designed to assist medical students in public hospitals in New Zealand with the diagnosis and treatment of patients. It was developed by the University of Otago School of Medicine, with a grant from the New Zealand Department of Health. It is an Internet-based system. The data in Mentor is based on 'competencies'. Students are presented with a list from which they select the presenting symptom. They work through the system by selecting items from a list that appears at each level. The system is primarily an information storage and retrieval system, with limited interactive capabilities and no modelling facility.

Information systems and decision support

Decision support systems couple the intellectual resources of individuals with the capability of the computer to improve the quality of decisions. It is a computer-based support system for management decision makers who deal with semi-structured problems (Gorry & Scott-Morton 1971).

The discipline of information systems views decision support systems as computer systems intended to assist decision-makers to use data, documents, knowledge, and/or models to identify problems and make decisions to resolve these. These systems are a particular type of information system comprising a data management system, a model management system, a knowledge-based management system, and the user interface:

- *Data management system*: DSS database (accessing internal and external data), a database management system that stores, retrieves data, and generates reports, a data dictionary that describes the data elements, and a query facility that enables questions to be asked of the DSS

- *Model management system*: standard models and models specifically written for the DSS
- *Knowledge-based management system*: consists of one or more intelligent systems that capture the expertise necessary for solving some aspects of the problem and supports the process of the decision-making
- *User interface*: provides a variety of input and output devices, output formats, dialogue styles, flexible and adaptive dialogue support and documentation.

These subsystems interact to produce the outputs that support the decision-making process.

Decisions may be structured, unstructured, or semi-structured. Structured decisions are those decisions made on a daily basis using well-established guidelines and static rules. These decisions are predictable and expected. Unstructured decisions are unique and often made in situations where alternatives and consequences are not known or clear. Semi-structured decisions are those where some but not all information is known.

Information systems falling under the umbrella of decision support range from a simple spreadsheet such as Excel, with its rudimentary decision support functionality, to complex systems that incorporate both the content and the process of reasoning in situations where there is a high degree of uncertainty. Table 9.1 lists categories of information systems considered to be decision support systems. For detailed information about different types of systems there are WWW links and references at the end of the chapter.

Table 9.1 Categories of decision support system

System	Application
Expert systems	Provide advice based on a knowledge database and models created through intensive input from experts
Artificial neural networks	Attempt to exhibit pattern recognition by learning from past experiences
Intelligent agents	Automate routine tasks to increase productivity and consistency
Knowledge management systems	Capture, store, and disseminate organisational knowledge
Executive information systems	Provide timely, summarised information through a graphical interface to executives
Group support systems	Support the processes of group work
Enterprise resource planning and supply chain management	Are closely related to decision support, customer relationship management, and e-commerce

The characteristics that see these systems categorised as decision support systems are summarised by Marakas (2003, p. 3). Decision support systems:

- are employed in semi-structured or unstructured decision contexts
- are intended to support decision makers rather than replace them
- support all phases of the decision-making process
- focus on the effectiveness of the decision-making process rather than its efficiency
- are under the control of the user
- use underlying data and models
- facilitate learning on the part of the decision maker
- are interactive and user-friendly
- are generally developed using an evolutionary, iterative process
- provide support for all levels of management from top executives to line managers
- can provide support for multiple independent or interdependent decisions
- provide support for individual, group, and team-based decision-making contexts.

The information systems view emphasises that, as with any other computer-based information system, the focus in decision support is not only on computers, but on the system as a whole. Therefore, when discussing the nature and application of decision support systems, the people, decisions, and the manner in which those decisions are made, must also be carefully assessed.

Knowledge-based or non-knowledge-based decision support

Decision support systems (DSSs) are information systems or knowledge-based systems designed to assist in the decision-making process. Information systems are non-knowledge-based systems that are used to manipulate data, which may sometimes be transformed into information for use in specific situations.

In a knowledge-based approach, knowledge is incorporated within the system. This allows the computer to 'think'. These systems are not intended to make decisions without human intervention, but rather to provide the tools and procedures to improve the quality of the user's decision-making process.

In health care, decision support systems have application in both the administrative and clinical environments.

Administrative decision support

Within the administrative environment, decision support systems are used to support semi-structured and unstructured managerial decisions, particularly at the senior executive level. Alter (1980) identified seven different categories of DSS based on the extent to which outputs provide direct support for a decision:

- *File drawer systems*: are the simplest type of decision support system. They provide access to data, which is then used to make a decision.
- *Data analysis systems*: have some data manipulation capabilities.
- *Analysis information systems*: provide access to multiple data sources, combine data from different sources, and enable data analysis.
- *Accounting models*: use internal accounting data and provide modelling capabilities. These systems cannot handle uncertainty.

- *Representational models*: can incorporate uncertainty and use models to solve decision problems using forecasting.
- *Optimisation models*: are used to estimate the effects of different decision alternatives.
- *Suggestion models*: are descriptive models used to suggest the best action. These may incorporate an expert system.

Alter proposed that these categories fell into two principal system orientations (data and models) and mapped them to common problem-solving and decision-making tasks—that is, operational, analysis, planning, budgeting, and resource allocation. Figure 9.1 synthesises the relationships among these tasks, components, and orientations.

Figure 9.1 Categories of administrative decision support system

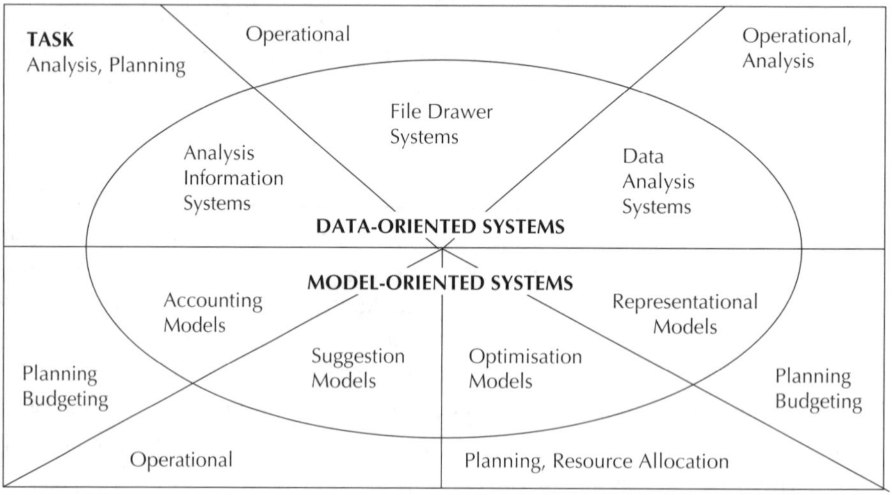

Source: adapted from Alter 1980

Health care organisations utilise commercial decision support systems to assist with strategic planning, finance, human resource management, service demand, and scheduling of personnel and facilities.

Clinical decision support

Diagnostic and other clinical support systems are a practical application of medical informatics (Carlson 1996).

Interest in clinical decision support systems (CDSSs) is not new. MYCIN, an expert system for diagnosing and recommending treatment for bacterial infections of the blood, was developed in the 1970s. Interest remains strong.

An investigation of electronic decision support initiatives in Australia identified 35 significant electronic decision support systems in routine use. Nearly half the projects are multi-state or national. While projects were identified in every state and Territory, the majority are situated in the more populous states (New South Wales and Victoria). Implementations were found predominantly in primary care (40 per cent) and hospital (28 per cent) settings (Sintechenko et al. 2002).

Yet, despite continuing interest, DSSs have been slow to achieve widespread acceptance or use in the clinical environment.

The promise of clinical decision support systems

> Medicine is a field in which help is critically needed. Our increasing expectations of the highest quality health care and the rapid growth of ever more detailed medical knowledge leave the physician without adequate time to devote to each case and struggling to keep up with the newest developments in his field. Most medical decisions must be based on rapid judgments of the case relying on the physician's unaided memory (Szolivits 1982).

The health care environment is characterised by information overload: 'It is estimated that we use nearly 2 billion pieces of information in our decision-making and that biomedical knowledge is doubling every twenty years' (Ramnarayan & Britto 2002, p. 361). Health professionals are expected to draw on this ever-increasing knowledge base in the daily process of diagnosing and treating patients. Yet this mass of information makes the selection of relevant information difficult, which could lead to clinicians overlooking or misinterpreting the data or information they elicit at the point of care.

Health professionals also draw on experience and expertise built up over years of clinical practice. Yet it is a characteristic of many health care systems that experience and expertise is organised in an inverted pyramid, with most wisdom concentrated among senior clinicians, who are often several steps removed from the patient. Consequently, expertise is not always available in the right place or at the right time. This too may contribute to errors or omissions in diagnosis and prescription.

Medical error is relatively common in the health care system, with the most common occurrence of medical errors taking place during the diagnostic and prescription phase of care. Since decision support systems are typically utilised at the point of care, their potential to reduce error is evident. Prevention of prescription error, in particular, is perceived as one of the most successful applications of clinical decision support systems (Trowbridge & Weingarten 2002).

Thus, the introduction of clinical decision support systems is expected to provide benefits in the related areas of improved patient safety, improved quality of care, and improved efficiency.

There is limited evidence to support these expectations and the quality of research around clinical decision support has been questioned. Critics observe that the number of rigorous studies are quite small, that the majority focus on user satisfaction with little attention given to evaluating patient outcomes or cost-effectiveness (as with so many other areas of health informatics), and that overall, the studies tend to be poorly conceptualised and implemented (Gawande & Bates 2000, Coiera 2004). However, published studies of CDSSs are increasing and it has been suggested that their quality is improving (Hunt et al 1998). While clinical decision support systems may live up to their promise in the future, the number of systems that have become integrated into everyday clinical care is still relatively small.

Applications of clinical decision support systems

Applications for decision support systems include:

- reminders and alerts
- prescribing systems
- diagnostic systems
- therapy critiquing and planning
- image recognition and interpretation.

Reminders and alerts

Reminders and alerts have application in both primary and tertiary environments. In primary care, information overload and time pressures may result in health professionals overlooking some relevant information during consultations. Reminders and alerts seek to address this by providing professionals with timely and patient-specific information during consultations. They can also act as prompts to remind clinicians of tasks—for example, immunisations that need to be carried out. In acute clinical environments, patient monitoring devices such as ECG can warn of changes in a patient's condition. Box 9.2 describes such a system.

BRIGHAM AND WOMEN'S HOSPITAL, BOSTON

The hospital has instituted an alert system whereby a computer constantly scans new data, including patient laboratory results as they are generated. If it encounters a critical value—for example, a substantial decrease in haemoglobin levels, or a dangerous potassium level—the computer will automatically page the patient's covering resident. If the resident does not respond within 15 minutes, the computer flashes a red alert signal for nurses on the patient's floor. If a nurse does not respond within 20 minutes, the computer phones a human dispatcher (Gawande & Bates 2000).

Prescribing systems

Prescribing systems check for drug–drug interactions, dosage errors, and other contraindications such as allergies. Box 9.3 describes a prescribing system, also from the Brigham and Women's Hospital.

BOX 9.3

PRESCRIBING SYSTEM

The system automatically suggests appropriate dosages to physicians and checks for drug allergies and drug–drug interactions. In its first year of use, this system resulted in a 55 per cent decrease in serious medication errors.

Diagnostic systems

Diagnostic systems have long been a focus of those interested in developing clinical decision support systems. The original concept was to develop a doctor-in-a-box, which would be so proficient at diagnosis that it would replace the clinician. Today, the focus is more on providing support to the clinician. Box 9.4 describes such a system.

BOX 9.4

DIAGNOSTIC SYSTEM

We developed a Bayesian network to assist with diagnosis of pulmonary embolism, including 72 variables to represent both the risk factors and the pathophysiological consequences of the disease. The network appears to be able to detect which observations make others irrelevant, so that decisions can be tailored to single cases (Luciani et al. 2003, p. 698).

Therapy critiquing and planning

Therapy critiquing and planning look for inconsistencies, errors and omissions in an existing treatment plan.

Image recognition and interpretation

Many clinical images can now be automatically interpreted. This is of value in mass screenings—for example, when the system can flag potentially abnormal images for detailed human attention. See Box 9.5.

These applications and examples demonstrate the varying levels of complexity of clinical decision support systems. The Australian National Institute for Clinical Studies has developed a four-scale classification system for electronic decision. The simpler, Type One, systems only provide categorised information that requires further processing and analysis by users before a decision can be made. The more complex systems are able to match characteristics of individual patients with a computerised knowledge base and generate patient-specific and situation-specific recommendations. Systems that generate conclusions from patient data typically utilise knowledge-based technologies. See Table 9.2.

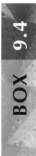

COMPUTER-BASED EXPERT ASSISTANCE FOR RADIOLOGISTS

The system identifies major structures in chest X-rays by comparing the imaged structures with a symbolic model of the anatomy of the chest. The size, locations, and appearance of structures are compared with normal values in the model, and discrepancies are reported as 'abnormalities' in a report designed to closely resemble a standard radiological report. The result is a system capable of providing decision support for less experienced clinicians (Wilson 1999).

Table 9.2 Classification system for decision support

Type	Explanation
Type One	Provides categorised information that requires further processing and analysis by users before a decision can be made.
Type Two	Presents the clinician with trends of patients' changing clinical status and alerts clinicians to out-of-range assessment results and intervention strategies. Clinicians are prompted to review information related to the alerts before arriving at a clinical decision.
Type Three	Uses deductive inference engines to operate on a specific knowledge base and automatically generates diagnostic or intervention recommendations based on changing patient clinical conditions, with the knowledge and inference engines stored in the knowledge base.
Type Four	Uses more complex knowledge management and inference models—such as case management reasoning, neural networks, or statistical discriminant analysis—to perform outcome or prognostic predictions. Such systems possess self-learning capabilities and use fuzzy set formalism and similarity measures or confidence level computation as mechanisms to deal intelligently and accurately with uncertainty.

Source: National Institute of Clinical Studies, 2002.

More complex clinical decision support systems are usually embedded in other computer applications, such as those used for prescribing and dispensing medicines, electronic health records, and other information systems used in health settings. Box 9.6 describes a complex system incorporating a number of systems, including clinical decision support.

BOX 9.6

UNIVERSITY OF ILLINOIS MEDICAL CENTER, CHICAGO

Several years ago, the 450-bed tertiary facility and major teaching hospital decided to implement a comprehensive electronic patient record and physician order entry system in both its inpatient and outpatient settings. Known as the Gemini Project, the initiative was designed to replace the medical center's obsolete, 15-year-old patient information software. Today, Gemini is operational and generating major benefits for the University of Illinois Medical Center (UIMC). Thanks to the system's electronic health record, more than two million patient records are now available electronically from 2800 personal computers located across the institution. The system's order entry system, meanwhile, has dramatically improved the speed and accuracy of orders ranging from medications to radiology reports. 'We couldn't be happier with how Gemini is working, and how well it's been embraced by our clinical staff,' said Joy Keeler, Associate Vice-Chancellor at UIMC. 'The most exciting thing is that we feel like we've only begun to realize the many benefits that Gemini can provide.' Dr George Kondos, an associate professor of medicine and the director of clinical cardiology at UIMC, says he believes Gemini has 'revolutionized' health care at the medical center. 'It's extremely efficient, it improves communications between the nursing staff, consulting physicians and the physician caring for the patient, and it provides for online access to test results,' said Kondos. 'We're getting up-to-date data that we used to have to wait hours and hours for.' The system's decision support capabilities—which alert clinicians to potential adverse drug interactions and patient allergies—has reduced the risks of mistakes in the administration of medications. A benefits study conducted in late 2000 by UIMC and Cerner concluded that, collectively, the Gemini applications already have produced savings of about $3.6 million at the medical center. Specific benefits revealed by the study include:

- With physicians accessing medical records from virtually anywhere in the institution, the medical center's house staff are now spending, on average, about 30 per cent less time looking for charts. That translates into about 30 minutes saved per day.
- Similarly, attending radiologists are spending, on average, five fewer hours per week reviewing medical records. The time savings is jointly attributable to easier film access as well as the ability to call up a patient's complete medical record electronically from the Gemini system.

- Registered nurses in the charge nurse role report spending 2.75 less hours per shift in the medication administration process, while nurses in the patient caregiver role report spending one less hour in the medication administration process.
- University of Illinois was so confident in the Gemini system that it designed and constructed a $100-million, 245 000-square-foot outpatient care center without any medical record storage space. The decision resulted in a one-time construction cost savings of $1.7 million, along with annual maintenance cost avoidance of $40 000.

Keeler says a host of other benefits continue to accrue. Before the installation of Gemini, the medical center estimated that a patient's paper record was unavailable when they arrived for care about 40 per cent of the time. Today, those records are accessible 100 per cent of the time for physicians, nurses, and other clinicians working across the care continuum.

Similarly, with UIMC's earlier, paper-based system, the average turnaround time before paper laboratory and radiology reports reached the physician was three days to one week. With Gemini, diagnostic test results are available within seconds of being verified, and are brought to the physician's attention through their desktop inbox to enable them to use this information in their decision-making. In addition, redundant orders that were often triggered by results delays have been virtually eliminated with the faster turnaround time and increased accessibility of the ubiquitous record. Duplicate checking on all orders placed in the system assists in controlling the costs of health care delivery. In addition, Gemini analyzes all medication orders for potential adverse drug interactions against patient allergies, other medications administered, as well as patient diets. 'In 2001 UIMC will be using information technology to continue to redesign health care delivery processes and assist clinicians in selecting the best treatment to be provided in a safe and effective manner,' according to Dr Anne LeMaistre, director of clinical systems. Already UIMC has explored the use of rules for improved care, but will be expanding their efforts using both ADE alerts and internally developed rules to support clinical decision-making.

As Kondos noted, communication between clinicians likewise has been vastly improved, particularly between the emergency room and primary care physicians. In fact, Kondos said, the overall increased efficiency that Gemini provides is allowing physicians to see more patients than they could before. Nurses, meanwhile, have reported saving time during their discussions with insurance companies. With the Gemini system, the patient information required is available on one screen. In the previous, main-frame–based, system nurses had to flip back and forth between multiple screens, a tedious task that cost them a considerable amount of time over the course of a day. Patients also have been saved time and aggravation, since the ubiquity of the desktop records means the patient is no longer asked the same questions numerous times by various caregivers throughout the institution. More importantly, patients benefit because caregivers have such complete and instant access to the patient's record. The result is faster, more effective, and more informed treatment. And despite initial scepticism by some staffers, Keeler said EMR usage levels at UIMC are now exceeding expectations, with more than 1600 caregivers accessing the system daily. Those using the system range from physicians to nurses to clerical staff. In February 2001, 481 617 total charts were opened, with peak usage of 7203 charts opened in a single day. On average, usage by position is about 40 per cent nurses, 36 per cent physicians, 10 per cent non-licensed clinical support, 5 per cent clerical staff, 5 per cent students and 4 per cent pharmacists.

'Our clinicians have embraced Gemini because it allows them to work faster and smarter,' Keeler said. 'With this foundation in place, we look forward to continuing to expand the functionality and power of Gemini, and will be placing a particular emphasis on decision support capabilities and transforming the remainder of the medical center in the months ahead.'

Source: adapted from 'University of Illinois Medical Center Chicago', used with permission from Cerner Corporation.

UNDERSTANDING CLINICAL DECISION SUPPORT SYSTEMS

Understanding clinical decision-making

Semi-structured decisions, where some but not all information is known, are the most common type of clinical decision. An example of this kind of situation was discussed in Chapter 2. It was explained that in a clinical situation a patient may complain of headache, shivering, abdominal pain, and vomiting. These symptoms, depending on their relative importance, will lead towards one diagnosis or another. The clinicians apply fuzzy logic in most clinical situations, producing a relative 'weighting' of symptoms, which is achieved by asking specific questions of the patient, by physical examination, or by clinical testing. The clinician might 'weight' the symptoms as shown in Table 9.3.

Table 9.3 Relative importance of symptoms

Symptom	Score (1 = high, 4 = low)					
Headache	1	4	1	3	3	4
Shivering	2	2	3	2	1	3
Abdominal pain	4	1	4	1	4	2
Vomiting	3	3	2	4	2	1
Suggested diagnoses (Table 9.4)	**A**	**B**	**C**	**D**	**E**	**F**

This would lead to a possible diagnosis, as seen in Table 9.4.

Table 9.4 Suggested diagnoses

Symptom score	Possible diagnoses
A	Meningitis, brain abscess, influenza
B	Appendicitis, right lower lobar pneumonia, cholecystitis, pancreatitis
C	Brain tumour, migraine, influenza
D	Influenza, diverticulitis, infectious mononucleosis
E	Malaria, influenza, dengue
F	Bowel obstruction, infectious mononucleosis

Note: This is an example and is not intended to be an accurate or realistic diagnosis.

Since decision support systems are intended to support decision makers through the decision-making process in semi-structured or unstructured situations, they appear to be particularly well suited to providing support for clinical decision-making. To effectively utilise decision support systems, however, we need to be able to identify, capture, manipulate, and represent expert clinical knowledge in ways that are both useful and acceptable to clinicians. This requires an understanding of knowledge and knowledge representation.

Understanding knowledge and knowledge representation

In Chapter 3, the distinction was made between explicit and tacit knowledge. Explicit knowledge can be further differentiated into descriptive and practical knowledge. Descriptive knowledge is knowledge about situations, conditions, events, people, and places. Practical knowledge is 'how to' knowledge and is often represented as a set of steps or instructions. These types of knowledge are easy to access and share through such mechanisms as formulae, protocols, care pathways, rules, and in databases. Tacit, or inferential knowledge is acquired through reasoning. Reasoning draws on other inferential knowledge, such as theory, and existing tacit knowledge to create new inferential knowledge. It is this form of knowledge that is the focus of knowledge-based clinical decision support systems, and which forms the basis of the inference process used in these systems.

Acquiring and representing inferential knowledge is a significant challenge for systems developers. Inferential knowledge is unstructured and loose, involving subjective insight, intelligence, and intuition. It is more difficult to communicate than is explicit knowledge because it resides in people's minds and they may not even have articulated it to themselves. It is therefore difficult to capture and format for use in computer systems. Various forms of knowledge representation and inference processes have been utilised to represent knowledge once it has been captured. These are discussed in the next section of the chapter.

An additional problem once knowledge has been 'captured' in a decision support system is maintaining the currency of that knowledge. New knowledge can quickly make redundant the existing knowledge base in a decision support system.

Understanding artificial intelligence

Until recently only a few intelligent systems achieved common clinical use (Begley et al. 2000, p. 1).

Since the 1970s, work on clinical decision support has occurred primarily within the field of artificial intelligence. Artificial intelligence has been a staple of science fiction since the 1920s, and a topic of intense debate in academic circles since the Second World War. See Box 9.7.

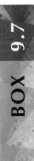

INTELLIGENT COMPUTERS?

BOX 9.7

In 1950, Alan Turing wrote a paper describing an experiment that he claimed could be used to test whether or not a computer is thinking. This has become known as the Turing Test. The test involves at least two humans and a computer, each of whom are kept separate from one another. One person asks the other person(s) and the computer a series of questions. The purpose of the questions is to try to discover which participant is the computer. If the questioner cannot do so, the computer is said to have passed the Turing Test and exhibited intelligence. There is ongoing debate about the validity of the Turing Test, yet the idea of an intelligent computer is still an intriguing one.

Approaches to intelligent systems

Within the field of AI, there are a number of different approaches to the development of an intelligent decision support system. Some of the more widely used of these are:

- expert systems
- belief networks
- neural networks
- fuzzy logic
- case-based reasoning.

Expert systems

Early researchers in artificial intelligence in medicine sought to develop AI systems that could make clinically accurate diagnoses. One of the earliest of these was MYCIN (1972–80), an interactive DSS that diagnosed infectious diseases and prescribed antimicrobial therapy. Although shown to rival the performance of health care specialists, MYCIN never became established as a routine tool. It did lead to the development of a large number of similar intelligent systems. A number of these, or their descendants, are still in use. Table 9.5 lists some early systems.

Table 9.5 Early expert systems

CDSS and its developers	Purpose
ABEL Massachusetts Institute of Technology	Acid-Base and Electrolyte expert system, employs causal reasoning to manage electrolyte and acid base derangements.
CASNET/Glaucoma Rutgers University	Used for diagnosis and treatment of glaucoma. Uses a causal-associational network model for describing disease process. Implemented in FORTRAN.
DeDombal's system Leeds University	Attempted to automate reasoning under uncertainty. Designed to support diagnosis of acute abdominal pain.
DXplain Laboratory of Computer Science, Massachusetts General Hospital, Harvard Medical School	Utilises clinical findings (signs, symptoms, laboratory data) to produce a ranked list of diagnoses that might explain (or be associated with) the signs or symptoms. It is currently used in the clinical and educational environment.
INTERNIST-I University of Pittsburgh	Used for diagnosis in general internal medicine. Deduces a list of compatible disease states from patient observations. Its medical knowledge base was used as a basis for successor systems (CADUCEUS and QMR).
MYCIN Stanford University	Used to diagnose and recommend treatment for blood infections and other infectious diseases. A goal-directed system that uses a backward chaining reasoning strategy. Was the predecessor to E-MYCIN, an expert system shell.

Table 9.5 Early expert systems (*cont.*)

CDSS and its developers	Purpose
ONCOCIN Stanford University	Developed at Stanford University, this system was designed to assist clinicians with the treatment of cancer patients receiving chemotherapy. One of the first systems that attempted to model decisions.
PUFF Stanford University and Pacific Presbyterian Medical Center	Probably the first AI system used in clinical practice. Used for interpretation of pulmonary function data. Commercial descendants are still used today.
QMR (Quick Medical Reference) University of Pittsburgh	A diagnostic decision-support system, developed at the University of Pittsburgh for interns to use as an electronic textbook, as a spreadsheet for diagnostic concepts and as an expert consultant program. The system uses clinical findings to describe the features of diseases listed in the QMR knowledge base. Windows versions of this system are currently available.

Source: adapted from Openclinical 2001.

Expert systems consist of three elements: a knowledge base, an inference engine, and a user interface.

The knowledge base

Expert systems manipulate expert knowledge, usually expressed in sets of 'if-then' rules, rather than data. The knowledge is obtained by interviewing people who are expert in the area in question. The interviewer or knowledge engineer organises this expert knowledge into a collection of rules, usually structured as 'if-then' statements. Box 9.8 is a sample interview, while Box 9.9 shows the knowledge structured as rules.

The inference engine

The inference engine manipulates the data by applying the rules. This enables the expert system to draw deductions from the rules in the knowledge base. This is shown in Box 9.10.

The user interface

This is the part of the system that interacts with the user. In the past, the user interface was not considered as part of the expert system technology so it was not given much attention. Awareness of software usability issues has brought about an understanding that the user interface can make a critical difference in the perceived utility of a system, regardless of how well that system performs.

BOX 9.8

ELICITING EXPERT KNOWLEDGE

Interviewer: With the colour of the dipstick, if we notice that...

Expert: Okay, well if it's darker, it's telling you that there are fairly significant levels of leucocytes in her urine. And you'd certainly want to investigate that a lot further.

Interviewer: All right, so what does...

Expert: Well, this is a fairly significant finding in pregnancy.

Interviewer: Right. So that would require attention?

Expert: It would require attention. Clearly immediate attention. It's not an urgent situation, but it would require...it needs treatment fairly quickly.

Interviewer: So, if you found leucocytes and it appeared to be a problem, what is the next thing you would do?

Expert: Well, I would question her once again—the same sort of questions that I would ask if I thought it was a urinary tract infection. Does she have pain on passing urine, what is the quality of the pain or the characteristics of the pain, um, and, if she described, for example, and I'm thinking of someone I interviewed just last week, if she described an intense burning, you'd really want to have a look at her genital area. Her vulva and around her urethra, because it will give you other information about the likelihood of a urinary tract infection or possibly a genital infection.

Interviewer: What other information?

Expert: If you noticed redness, or she, or possibly you might even notice, um, pustules, or raw areas, ulcerations on her skin, that might tell you that she doesn't actually have a urinary tract infection, but that she is more likely to have a genital infection and simply the burning of the urine may not be the fact that the urine is infected, but the fact that the acid of the urine is passing over a raw area and is proving very painful.

Interviewer: Good. When you say redness, how red is redness?

BOX 9.9

IF-THEN STATEMENTS

If dipstick = pink, THEN leucocytes = 0

If leucocytes = 0, THEN result = normal

If dipstick = lilac and symptoms = none, THEN result = normal

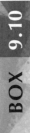

IF-THEN RULES FOR AN EXPERT SYSTEM

BOX 9.10

If dipstick = high, and temperature = high, and micturition = pain, THEN result = problem.

If result = problem, and pain = kidney area, and vulva = itch, THEN problem = kidney infection.

Knowledge-based systems have had some acceptance as clinical decision-support tools, but this has been within limited areas. Shortcomings include:

- Extracting knowledge from a human expert can be very difficult.
- Larger systems require a large number of rules.
- Expert systems tended to focus on a narrow area of clinical knowledge.
- Since medical knowledge is constantly changing, it is difficult to maintain the currency of the knowledge base.
- Systems often need to ask a great number of questions to obtain the information needed to draw conclusions.
- Clinicians resist using systems that are time consuming and difficult to use.

Belief networks

Belief networks are also known as Bayesian belief networks. They are named after the Reverend Thomas Bayes who reportedly developed a probabilistic theorem (1763) in an attempt to prove the existence of God (Ramnarayan & Britto 2002, p. 361). The theorem is used in belief networks to calculate updated disease probabilities as new evidence (say a test result, for example) becomes available and is analysed in the context of background information (prevalence of disease). The system diagnosing pulmonary embolism (PE) described in Box 9.4 was a Bayesian network. It 'consists of 72 nodes representing PE associated clinical events and several medical hypotheses commonly involved in the medical diagnosis' (Luciani et al. 2003). One disadvantage of Bayesian systems is that it is necessary to know probability distributions in order to create a system. Luciani et al. 'retrieved the quantitative measures of associations from the literature through a critical review of available studies and agreement on the assumptions made to cope with the lack of published information' (2003, p. 698). This is clearly an involved and time-consuming process.

Neural networks

A neural network is a computer-based modelling technique that is intended to operate the way a human brain does. Neural networks usually consist of several layers of neurons with interconnections between the nodes in each layer. Figure 9.2 models a simple neural network.

Figure 9.2 Neural network

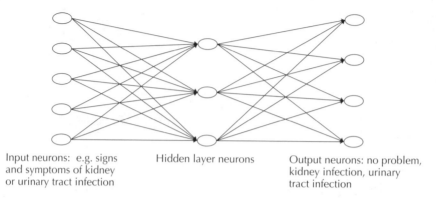

Input neurons: e.g. signs
and symptoms of kidney
or urinary tract infection

Hidden layer neurons

Output neurons: no problem,
kidney infection, urinary
tract infection

Neural networks are not programmed or knowledge engineered. Rather, they are 'trained' to recognise specific patterns as data is entered. Box 9.11 describes the 'training' process.

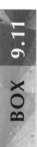

TRAINING THE NEURAL NETWORK

The model is trained by using data from a representative population with defined input variables and a known outcome variable. After iterative training, the network is tested in another population with the same input variables, but during testing, the network is blinded to the outcome variable.

Fuzzy logic

Often, when attempting to gather knowledge for an expert system, the knowledge engineer finds that human experts use vague or ambiguous expressions. This is particularly the case with clinical knowledge. Ambiguous expressions are difficult to deal with in standard logic, which has only two values: true and false.

Fuzzy logic attempts to deal with reasoning using ambiguous terms. It seeks to differentiate degrees of certainty and uncertainty.

Case-based reasoning

Case-based reasoning assumes that new problems are often similar to previously encountered problems, and that those previously successful solutions, or adaptations of these, may be applicable to the current situation. CDSSs using case-based reasoning contain a library of cases, rather than knowledge represented by rules. Each case includes a description of the problem and solution or outcome. The system works by matching new problems to 'cases' from the library and then adapting successful solutions from the past to current situations. These are tried and revised or adapted if necessary. The new problem and solution are then included in the library of cases.

ISSUES

> While there certainly have been ongoing challenges in developing such systems, they actually have proven their reliability and accuracy on repeated occasions (Shortliffe 1989). Much of the difficulty experienced in introducing them has been associated with the poor way in which they have fitted into clinical practice, either solving problems that were not perceived to be an issue, or imposing changes in the way clinicians worked (Coiera 2003, p. 332).

Despite the apparent success of a number of clinical decision support systems, they have had a relatively limited impact in mainstream clinical care. A number of reasons have been identified for this. As with many other applications of health informatics, many of these reasons stem from the organisational and cultural aspects of health care, rather than from the technology used to develop CDSSs. There are, however, some issues relating to the technology.

Technology issues

As with many areas where technology is used for the storage and exchange of clinical information, standards are an issue. As with electronic health records, vocabularies to ensure common use and understanding of concepts are an important issue for clinical decision support. The case study on University of Illinois Medical Center (Box 9.6) pointed to the potential for integrating decision support with other clinical and administrative systems. To facilitate this, while also protecting PID, relevant standards must be implemented.

Safety is a significant issue for clinical information systems. Safety issues range from minimising human error when entering data to questions of incorrect diagnosis or advice from a system. The safety standard IEC 61508 can be used as a basis for establishing best practice in the design and development of safety-critical systems.

The nature of clinical knowledge

The discussion in an earlier section of this chapter highlighted the difficulties around capturing clinical knowledge. Most decision support systems deal with only a narrow field, and even within their identified domain, only part of the relevant knowledge can be conceptualised in a usable form. Intuitive diagnostic processes, many of which are unique to the individual clinician, cannot be transferred to a machine. Nor can the social and psychological problems that are so frequently an element of human illness. The use of clinical decision support systems may therefore result in an emphasis on physical symptoms and laboratory data, with social and psychological information being neglected. This presents the possibility of a shift from patient-centred to disease-centred care (Marckmann 2001).

Professional roles

The protocols involved, and the need to enter and access information into clinical decision support systems, may require changes in workflow and routines. While systems developers are becoming more aware of the need to integrate CDSSs into clinical workflow, many current systems still require the clinician to enter patient information by typing or selecting from a range of options. This may be time consuming and disruptive to the normal work flow. Integration of CDSSs into other clinical systems is one solution being considered. Linking to an electronic health record, for example, would 'allow decision support to occur in the background, the system extracting patient details from the EPR and delivering patient-specific advice to the user at appropriate points' (Ramnarayan & Britto 2002).

Patient–clinician relationships

The centrality of the patient–clinician relationship, particularly the face-to-face consultation, has been highlighted previously. CDSSs have the potential to be perceived as dehumanising patient care through an emphasis on the technology. This may be particularly so if the CDSS requires the attention of the clinician to enter data and information, or if the system is perceived as fulfilling a doctor-in-a-box role. On the other hand, CDSSs may facilitate efficient access to information, leaving clinicians more time to build caring relationships with their patients (Marckmann 2001).

Whatever view is held, it is clear that the acceptance of clinical decision support systems will be influenced by the extent to which they are perceived to support the patient–clinician relationship.

What decisions are CDSSs supporting?

There is general agreement that one of the key obstacles to the adoption of CDSSs relates to the types of decisions they are designed to support (Coiera 2004, Nykanen 2003, Shortliffe 1989). There has traditionally been a strong focus on developing CDSSs to assist with diagnoses. Heathfield and Wyatt (1993), for example, found that 53 per cent of available systems dealt with diagnostic problems, while only 19 per cent of systems dealt with therapy planning problems. Diagnosis, however, may comprise only a small part of what health professionals do in their daily practice. Altman (1997) suggests that many consultations are for an existing or previously diagnosed problem, and that health professionals really need support with following chronic and slowly evolving diseases. This is consistent with the observations made in Chapter 1 of increases in cardiovascular diseases, stress-related diseases, diabetes, and obesity in Western society, and increasing numbers of older consumers with multiple, chronic, and evolving health issues. It is also reflected in the Heathfield and Wyatt study, which found that only 6 per cent of the help queries to the Medline databases sought diagnostic support, while 41 per cent asked for help with therapy planning problems.

There appears to be a mismatch between the problems clinicians need help with, and the problems CDSSs are designed to provide assistance with. As Coiera (2004) notes, 'one of the most important tasks now facing the developers of AI-based systems is to characterise accurately those aspects of clinical practice that are best suited to the introduction of artificial intelligence systems.'

SUMMARY

Decision support, particularly clinical decision support, has been an area of interest since health informatics first began to emerge as a distinct discipline. Despite this, decision support systems have yet to impact significantly on main stream health care. This is attributable to the way in which the field of decision support has evolved, and also to the characteristics of the health care environment.

The field of decision support systems in health has been influenced by the disciplines of artificial intelligence and information systems. The field of artificial intelligence is concerned with the study of intelligent behaviour and knowledge engineering to create systems that mimic human intelligence. The two branches of AI are strong AI, which is based on the premise that computers can be made to think on a level equal to humans, and weak AI, which takes the view that some thinking-like functions can be programmed into computers to support human decision-making. Early work in clinical decision support was within the field of strong AI, and this resulted in an early technological focus.

The discipline of information systems approaches decision support from the perspective that decision support systems are computer systems intended to assist decision-makers to use data, documents, knowledge, and models to identify and resolve problems. Decision support systems comprise a data management system, a knowledge-based management system, a model management system and a user interface. These sub-systems interact to produce the outputs that support the decision-making process. Decisions may range from structured decisions that use well-established guidelines to unstructured decisions where alternatives and consequences are not known or clear. Within the health care environment, decision support primarily facilitates semi-structured decisions where some, but not all information is known.

Decision support systems can use either a non-knowledge-based or a knowledge-based approach. A non-knowledge-based approach involves the manipulation of data, whereas a knowledge-based approach draws on knowledge built into the system.

Within the administrative environment, commercial decision support systems assist with decisions in areas such as strategic planning, finance, human resource management, service demand, and scheduling. Clinical decision support systems offer the promise of enhancing clinical decision-making at the point of care by enabling enhanced access to relevant biomedical knowledge and the accumulated experience of expert clinicians. This, it is anticipated, will result in the reduction of errors and improved patient safety, quality of care, and efficiency. The main areas of application are for reminders and alerts, prescribing, diagnosis, therapy planning, and image recognition and interpretation.

Effective utilisation of clinical decision support systems requires the identification, capture, manipulation, and representation of expert knowledge in ways that are both useful and acceptable to clinicians. This requires an understanding of knowledge and knowledge representation. Knowledge can be defined as factual and explicit or tacit and inferential. The knowledge that occurs when understanding is applied to information is inferential and/or tacit knowledge. This is the form of knowledge that is the focus of knowledge-based clinical decision support systems and that forms the basis of the inference process used in these systems. Acquiring and representing this knowledge is one of the challenges for developers of decision support systems. Since we do not know how knowledge is represented in the human mind, and do not fully understand the human decision-making process, various forms of knowledge representation and inference processes are used. These include rule-based systems, statistical probability systems, neural networks, and fuzzy logic.

Expert systems are one of the most common types of clinical decision support systems. While these have had some acceptance, they also have a number of limitations, including the narrow range of clinical knowledge they can incorporate, the difficulty in maintaining the currency of medical knowledge, and cumbersome user interfaces.

Despite the apparent success of many clinical decision support system projects, they have had a limited impact in mainstream clinical care. Reasons for this include the limitations of systems with regard to capturing and depicting medical knowledge, the relevance of the decision support offered, and their impact on work routines, role, and relationships.

WWW LINKS

Expert systems

Friedman-Hill (1997), Hart (1986), Kandel (1992), Rolston (1988), Hayes-Roth et al. (1983), 'Expert systems' <http://www.aaai.org/AITopics/html/expert.html>

Intelligent agents

Agents 101, 'Start here to learn about agents' <http://agents.umbc.edu/>

Knowledge management systems

Alavi, M. 2004 'Knowledge management and knowledge management systems' <http://www.mbs.umd.edu/is/malavi/icis-97-KMS/>

Bellinger, G, 2004, 'Knowledge management: emerging perspectives' <http://www.systems-thinking.org/kmgmt/kmgmt.htm>

Executive information systems

Compinfo.ws <http://www.compinfo-center.com/entsys/executive_information_systems.htm>

Enterprise resource planning

Koch, C. 2002, 'The ABCs of ERPs', CIO.com <http://www.cio.com/research/erp/edit/erpbasics.html>

Safety

Fox, J. & Thomson, R. 2002, 'Clinical decision support systems: A discussion of quality, safety and legal liability issues' <http://www.acl.icnet.uk/lab/PUBLICATIONS/ms380.doc>

Morris, A.H. 2002, 'Decision support and safety of clinical environments' <http://qhc.bmjjournals.com/cgi/content/full/11/1/69>

CRITICAL THINKING

1 Research the issue of error in clinical decision support systems. How significant is this issue?
2 Use the interview in Table 9.8 to develop some IF-THEN rules, and some THEN applications of those rules.
3 How might clinical decision support systems be used without changing the patient focus of health care?
4 What areas of clinical decision-making are suited to the use of clinical decision support systems?

PART 3

HEALTH INFORMATICS IN ACTION

The potential of health informatics to enhance health care services, and the issues facing the field in attempting to do so, are best illustrated in a practical situation.

This last part of the book contains one chapter that seeks to demonstrate the use of health informatics in the real world. Chapter 10 focuses on the use of information management and communications tools and strategies in the rural and remote health care environment. Equity of access to health services in rural and remote areas has been an ongoing issue facing many health care providers around the world. Health informatics is seen as offering the capacity to provide some solutions to the problems of accessibility, quality, and cost of medical care.

This chapter uses a case-study approach to explore the issues and opportunities.

CHAPTER 10

HEALTH INFORMATICS IN ACTION: RURAL AND REMOTE HEALTH

OVERVIEW

The potential for health informatics to enhance health care services, and the issues faced in attempting to do so, are best illustrated using real-life examples. This enables an analysis of the complex social, political, and economic issues that impact on the health care environment. The provision of services to rural and remote areas is one area where the use of health information and communication systems have long been viewed as having considerable potential. These systems have the capacity to provide some solutions to the problems of accessibility, quality, and cost of medical care. In reality, the application of health informatics tools and systems, particularly for clinical consultations, is limited. It takes time to address access to appropriate and affordable infrastructure, ethical and medico-legal matters, security, and universal recognition of medical registration, high telecommunications costs, and issues of reimbursement for private practitioners for the provision of e-health services. These are the socio-technical issues of health informatics.

OBJECTIVES

- to demonstrate the application of health informatics in real communities
- to explore issues around the delivery of health care to rural and remote communities
- to examine those aspects of health informatics (tools, systems, and applications) with the capacity to enable better health outcomes for people in rural and remote regions
- to illustrate a health informatics approach to rural health through a case study of several projects.

CONCEPTS

Rural
Remote

INTRODUCTION

This chapter illustrates the application of health informatics by considering projects introduced by a regional health service in Australia. Rural health is an appropriate choice, since equity of access to health services in rural and remote areas has long been an issue for health care providers around the world, and health informatics systems have long been seen as the means to provide some solutions to these problems. To provide a context for the discussion, the chapter first outlines the broad challenges facing rural and remote communities. This discussion touches briefly on the complexities of terminology, definitions and classifications. The chapter then details the efforts of the regional health service to meet some of the demands for service delivery through use of information and communications systems. The chapter focuses on the Australian experience, enabling you to analyse the interplay between the specific social, economic, and political factors shaping health issues and health systems. The projects and situations discussed are actual events, but the identifying details have been omitted to enable a focus on the issues. The chapter concludes by considering the potential of health informatics as a planning tool at the strategic level.

THE CONTEXT

This section establishes the context by focusing on rural health, which is itself a complex area of study. The discussion of the area is necessarily brief. WWW links at the end of the chapter, and references at the end of the book, provide more in depth analyses of the field of rural health.

Defining rural

There is no standard definition of 'rural' used in policy, research, or planning. A multitude of terms are used interchangeably, both within the health care and in other sectors. Different definitions and classifications are used for different purposes and in different contexts. Many definitions, in addition to distinguishing between rural and urban, also acknowledge that 'remote' has its own unique characteristics and issues. Classifying degrees of remoteness is yet another area of discussion. There are, for example, three major remote classifications currently used in Australia. These are:

- Rural, Remote and Metropolitan Areas (RRMA)
- Accessibility/Remoteness Index of Australia (ARIA) based on ARIA index values
- Australian Standard Geographical Classification (ASGC) Remoteness Areas (based on ARIA + index values).

In Australia, as in many countries, rural is often defined in the context of exclusion. Everything outside the capital cities and major metropolitan centres is defined as rural. The existence of multiple classifications of remoteness, however, emphasises that there is no neat definition of rural that can be applied to all areas that are 'not in capital cities or metropolitan areas', just as there is no neat, precise definition of metropolitan that adequately describes the many locations falling within the parameters of metropolitan. Acknowledging the diversity and heterogeneity of rural and remote communities, and the similar differentiation of their health status, is fundamental to understanding and promoting rural and remote health. It is this diversity that should drive policy and planning, including the resourcing of health information and communications systems.

Rural health status

People living in rural and remote regions face many challenges, including health disadvantage. Research generally points to a progressive worsening in health status as population density and infrastructure decrease. At the same time, the standard stereotypes and generalisations about rural health may not always be accurate. Recent decades have seen population patterns becoming more diverse and complex, and much less predictable. The composition of rural populations has also become more heterogeneous. Just as rural and remote communities are heterogenous and diverse, so too are the health issues they face. The fact remains, however, that people living in rural and remote communities do share a number of health concerns and issues.

Policy makers, politicians, researchers, and community members are interested in the way people's lives vary according to where they live. In Australia, as in other countries, there is concern about the difficulties non-metropolitan communities have in accessing services. In particular, there is concern about possible differences in health, education, and income between those living in, and those living outside, metropolitan areas. This is acknowledged by governments and health services, which are, as Box 10.1 indicates, increasingly viewing rural health as a significant issue.

BOX 10.1

FOCUS ON RURAL HEALTH CARE

Australia

In 1994, the Commonwealth, state and rerritory Health Ministers jointly endorsed a National Rural Health Strategy (*Healthy Horizons*) to provide a coordinated framework for ensuring equitable access to effective health care for rural and remote communities through the provision of appropriate health services, the promotion of measures designed to maximise the health status of rural and remote residents, and the adoption of strategies that minimise barriers and problems that impede the delivery of effective care (AHMAC 2003). In 2004, the Strategy was reviewed (*Healthy Horizons: Outlook 2003–2007*), giving emphasis to contemporary issues, challenges, and emerging priorities, including developments in medical knowledge and technology and a primary health care approach.

New Zealand

In 2004, the New Zealand government's policy for rural health services focuses on the commitment by government and rural communities to maintaining and improving access to good-quality health and disability support services. The emphasis is on rural people and rural communities first, to create opportunities to develop local arrangements to meet their needs. It specifically focuses on the use of technology where possible to reduce the impact of isolation.

Canada

In Canada, rural health is gaining public attention with the development of special programs in almost all provinces and territories to address rural health issues—particularly rural physician shortages—and the creation of the Office of Rural Health within Health Canada. In 2002, a new federal Ministerial Advisory Committee on rural health was created and a significant number of rural health-related projects were initiated by the Health Transition Fund, which have been synthesised to generate a series of overarching policy-related recommendations (Health Canada 2002).

USA

The Office of Rural Health Policy (ORHP) was established in 1987 by the administration to inform and advise the Department of Health and Human Services on matters affecting rural hospitals and health care. It works within government at federal, state, and local levels and with the private sector to seek solutions to rural health care problems. There is a clear trend in the USA of policy efforts to pull health care providers into systems of health care delivery. The federal government has invested directly in local rural health projects through the outreach Grant Program, a 10-year commitment to rural communities, administered by the ORHP (Loue & Quill 2001).

In Australia, there are seven National Health Priority Areas, which focus on the diseases and conditions that cause the highest morbidity and mortality in the population. These include chronic illnesses that pose a significant health burden, and conditions that have potential for health gains and improved health outcomes:

- mental health
- diabetes
- cardiovascular health
- arthritis and musculoskeletal conditions
- injury prevention and control

- cancer control
- asthma (Department of Health and Ageing 2002).

Many of these health issues are exacerbated in rural and remote areas due to a range of factors including:

- difficulties attracting and retaining health workers
- high and increasing rates of diabetes among Aboriginal and Torres Strait Islander people
- very high rates of rheumatic fever and rheumatic heart disease among Aboriginal and Torres Strait Islander people
- lack of access to timely treatment in emergency situations
- lack of access generally to specialised services providing acute care, rehabilitation, and secondary prevention interventions
- difficulties instigating prevention programs in communities with poor access to fresh food.

Rural and remote communities also have health concerns that are not national health priority areas. Issues of healthy ageing, support for children and young people, addressing substance abuse, oral health, and overweight and obesity, have been identified as needing special attention, and the Australian National Public Health Partnership Framework is developing strategies to improve health across many issues and population groups in rural and remote Australia (AHMAC 2003). Discussion in publications such as *The New Rural Health* (Wilkinson & Blue 2002) and *Australia's Rural and Remote Health* (Smith 2004a) emphasise that this will best be achieved by establishing rural health as multidisciplinary and collaborative, with a strong population health focus.

Rural health systems

In Chapter 1 characteristics of contemporary health systems were identified as:

- knowledge- and technology-intensive biomedical model
- specialisation and differentiation
- bureaucratic structures
- health care structured around the face-to-face consultation.

These characteristics manifest in rural health systems in particular ways.

Knowledge- and technology-intensive biomedical model

The biomedical model with its focus on acute health issues has impacted significantly on rural health services. The increasingly sophisticated interventions and treatments are often very expensive and health systems are rationalising these to larger population centres to enable economies of scale. The need to access these services increasingly creates burdens for the consumer, who is required to travel to larger population centres for consultations.

Specialisation and differentiation

The silo models of health care used in urban areas are generally replicated in rural and remote areas. Access to specialist services also becomes increasingly difficult as these often expensive services are centralised to facilitate efficiencies. Professions intent on protecting their areas of expertise have exacerbated the problems. An example is the situation where prescriptions can only be written by a GP. If no GP is available, patients will be unable to get the prescriptions they need. As many rural and remote communities have fallen below the threshold for maintaining existing health services, silos are being increasingly challenged. There is increasing acceptance that rural health should be approached from a multidisciplinary, collaborative perspective (Wilkinson & Blue 2002, Smith 2004a).

Bureaucratic structures

The bureaucratic structures adopted by health systems encourage fragmentation across a range of programs and services. This makes local coordination of services difficult. It is not helpful to conceptualise rural and remote health as a system of vertical programs. Successful health services should be part of the horizontal integration of a range of sectors and services across communities.

Health care structured around the face-to-face consultation

The centrality of the face-to-face situation creates pressure for health professionals across the health system. It is exacerbated in rural areas as numbers of health professionals decline. The centrality of face-to-face consultations with specialists, generally located in larger population centres, creates issues of travel, time, and expense for consumers. The need to travel to attend pre-admission clinics is one example.

Issues for rural health systems

As with the broader health environment, these characteristics create issues for rural health services around maintaining services and managing clinical and health information.

Maintaining services

Until recently rural health services were structured around a network of small local hospitals. This model developed very early in our history when it was both possible and desirable to have duplication of a range of services and facilities. Medical care was much less complex and less technology dependent, and small rural hospitals were able to cope with most medical situations without demanding huge resources This was desirable at a time when the horse was the main form of transport, and not to have facilities dotted across the landscape would have meant grave danger for the seriously ill or injured individual more than a day's ride away from assistance.

Over the years the 'march of progress' has seen cheaper, faster, more efficient transport emerge, while commercial, education, and health services in rural communities have diminished or disappeared. Populations in rural communities have also declined. The combination of declining rural populations and the increasing rationalisation of expensive and complex treatments to larger centres has seen a decline in health services in rural and remote areas.

As communities and services decline, the recruitment and retention of suitably qualified clinicians and other health professionals becomes increasingly difficult. Reasons for this include:

- personal and family issues with living in a rural area, such as schooling, opportunities for partner employment, spectrum of social/leisure activities
- professional work satisfaction as opportunities for specialisation and career advancement are limited by low case numbers and critical mass of other specialists
- clinical risk, with low patient numbers and a requirement to work outside areas of expertise, which may expose clinicians to managing situations they are not competent to deal with (the risk is further enhanced by the increasingly litigious health environment)
- the potential for being almost continuously on-call
- less chance for continuing professional education because of remoteness
- less chance for involvement in teaching and research
- discrepancies in remuneration.

Yet small communities are surviving and many are becoming increasingly resentful of the gradual removal of services they have come to take for granted.

Managing information

The importance of information management is magnified in rural health because of the nature of dispersed populations and the issue of timely access to specialist medical and other health and related services. Rural health professionals often work in isolation and a health informatics approach to health care has the potential to lessen this isolation by providing an evidence base and decision support to improve practice.

Management of day-to-day health information, where such information may need to be communicated across geographically dispersed facilities, is a particular issue for rural health services. Issues of timely, accurate, and secure information sharing are magnified.

The Australian political and fiscal context

In Australia, political tensions between all levels of government—local, state and territory, federal and international—are drivers of change, and by their very nature are unpredictable. Medicare agreements, workforce responsibility (the medical workforce is currently a federal concern, while the nursing and oral health workforce is a state/ territory concern), responsibility for health, transport, and communications services, and corporatisation of health all reflect, and are influenced by, ongoing political tensions. Fiscal matters encompass not only the problem of fiscal constraints, but also fiscal coordination and rationing of health services. Fiscal issues are compounded by the known inflexibility of the health care system. It is becoming more and more expensive to deliver health care, particularly to rural and remote communities.

In recent years there has been increasing pressure on health service providers to exercise fiscal austerity and yet maintain, if not improve, the quality of health care offered to consumers. Health service providers are faced with the prospect of either cutting back on services, particularly in rural and remote communities where economies of scale are not possible, or facing huge increases in the demand for services and consequently in costs.

Information and communications systems are increasingly being heralded as one solution to the problems of accessibility, quality, and cost of providing services for rural and remote communities. In reality, the actual use of information and communications systems, particularly for clinical consultations, is limited as many issues, including appropriate and affordable infrastructure, medico-legal matters, and problems of medical registration and reimbursement are still to be addressed. The trend is increasingly towards the use of information and communications systems as a means of resolving some of the issues around providing health services to rural and remote communities and individuals.

INTRODUCING HEALTH INFORMATICS

This section describes health informatics projects initiated by a regional department of health within an Australian state. The projects sought to meet some challenges of delivering health care to rural and remote regions. While the situations and experiences are real, they have been de-identified to facilitate a focus on the programs and issues, which are shared by many organisations.

The region

The population in the region is widely dispersed. The large number of people living in small towns or rural locations away from the three regional centres makes it one of the most rural in Australia. This is part of the attraction for residents, particularly retirees who migrate to the region to enjoy the pleasures of living in small, friendly, rural communities, while never being more than a few hours away from a major centre. Rural health professionals also enjoy the small community feel of the region in their work environments. However, as with rural health professionals everywhere, they find that limited resources are making it increasingly difficult to maintain services. In common with worldwide trends there are increasing costs and complexities in delivering health services in the region, and services are becoming increasingly restricted because of isolation or distance from regional centres, the cost of providing regular visiting specialist and ancillary services, and a lack of health professionals available in the rural areas. The pressures to resolve these problems are as great, if not greater, than elsewhere in Australia because the population is ageing more rapidly, and because the cost of providing services is proportionately greater due to diseconomies of scale and the difficulties in serving a dispersed population.

The health service

Australian model

The regional department is part of the Australian health system and is therefore subject to the funding arrangements, health insurance, and reimbursement systems, and mix of public, private, and not-for-profit services of that system. These were discussed in Box 1.3 in Chapter 1.

The regional health system

This regional organisation was introduced in Box 3.7 in Chapter 3 as an example of a contemporary health care organisation. It is a large, complex organisation providing services across a wide geographical area encompassing both the urban environments of the regional centres and rural and remote communities. It employs 8500 people located within four sections spread across more than 300 sites. Each of the four sections focuses on a specific service area. Figure 10.1 depicts this structure.

Figure 10.1 The organisation structure

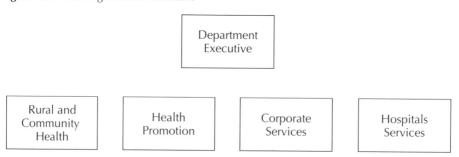

Broad responsibilities of each section are:

- *Corporate Services:* provides integrated internal support services across the organisation; establishes and oversees the implementation of organisation-wide policies and procedures
- *Health Promotion:* delivers a range of community and public programs directed to the promotion and protection of the health and well-being of citizens.
- *Rural and Community Health:* provides planning and coordination of services delivered in community and rural areas
- *Hospitals Services:* provides hospital and ambulance services and support for teaching and research.

The organisation is characterised by the typical, complex hierarchical structure of the contemporary health system. Decision-making on issues affecting the organisation as a whole is centralised. Section managers exercise a degree of autonomy within their own area. The two sections most affected by the health informatics projects are Hospitals Services and Rural and Community Health. Hospitals Services is structured around the traditional biomedical hierarchy, exhibiting the typical biomedical culture of strong professional boundaries between subcultures. This section deals with 'patients'. Rural and Community Health reflects the flatter, more democratic management structures that have been emerging in recent years. This division deals with 'clients' and 'consumers'. There is potential for misunderstanding and tension between health professionals in the two divisions.

The mid-1990s saw significant budget restrictions and a shift in resources away from service delivery to corporate services, and from community-based services to the acute care program. Many services to rural and remote communities were reduced or withdrawn. The closure of rural hospitals is one of the best publicised examples.

Frequent staff reductions and funding cuts have resulted in a degree of insecurity and conservatism across the organisation. There is a general reluctance to take risks and a degree of scepticism regarding change. There is a belief that change will result in either more staff reductions or increased workloads, or both. There is also a degree of demoralisation as staff are constantly expected to do more and more with less and less. Staff in Hospitals Services have suffered the majority of redundancies and are particularly sensitive to changes or initiatives that might further erode their resource base or increase their workload.

The potential of health informatics

During the 1990s the regional health department, as with health organisations everywhere, faced limited resources but escalating demands for services. Senior management recognised the potential of health informatics and made a broad decision to enhance health services through the development of a number of projects. These included:

- a roll-out of region-wide technology infrastructure
- the introduction of the health informatics education program
- the establishment of a telehealth network.

A community client management system was conceived and planned at a later date. This latter initiative is intended to link into a state-wide system, and ultimately interact with the Australian government Health*Connect* initiatives.

The projects

Technology infrastructure roll-out

In 1999, the technological capability of the regional health department was at an embryonic stage. Box 10.2 describes this capability.

This is typical, as reported by McGill in Chapter 1, in that 'spending on IT was much greater at the non-solutions, ad-hoc projects level rather than at the total solutions/strategic spending level' (McGill 2001, p. 2).

At the time, state and federal governments were encouraging the development of information and communications technology, and the regional health department had been promised significant funding to develop its regional infrastructure. This roll-out

BOX 10.2

TECHNOLOGICAL CAPABILITY

The technological capability of the regional health department is described below.

- There was no clear IT policy or strategy.
- A position for an IT manager existed, but no permanent appointment had been made.
- The agency was operating on a narrow bandwidth LAN (64KB ISDN to most connected sites) that was being heavily utilised. This resulted in unreliable access. Many rural and remote sites did not have any connection to the Intranet, or the Internet.
- The organisation was top heavy with desktop technology and under-resourced as far as networking was concerned.
- Desktop hardware and software were mixed, ranging from the latest Pentium-class machines and software to 386 computers running on Windows 3.1.
- New IT projects were implemented without regard to what was happening in other parts of the organisation, resulting in duplication and incompatibilities. This is typical of the silo development of information systems discussed in Chapter 6.

of infrastructure was clearly a key enabling tool for subsequent initiatives. Unfortunately a change of state government resulted in a scaling down of promised funds for the regional roll-out. At the same time the IT section of the department announced that the emphasis for the next two years was to be on financial management systems, rather than on systems to support health care delivery. A significant scaling down of the planned technology infrastructure roll-out resulted. Three years later, some rural and remote sites were only just being connected to the network.

Health informatics education program

Senior management were aware that use of the new information systems would be facilitated if staff had the skills to use them as they became available. An in-service education program was instituted. The program was to be online and offered in conjunction with the infrastructure roll-out. Content and format were to be based on needs assessments and surveys conducted during the early stages of the program. A collaborative arrangement was entered into with a regional training institution. This institution managed and implemented the program as a series of modules released over the life of the project. A project advisory committee consisted of four members of the training institution and three department representatives: two middle managers from IT and the manager of the telehealth project. The group met monthly, but attendance was sporadic. Box 10.3 summarises key elements of the project.

HEALTH INFORMATICS EDUCATION PROGRAM

- The project adopted a broad socio-technical education and training approach rather than a skills development approach linked to any specific project.
- The target group was primarily Hospitals Services, and Rural and Community Health, but staff from other sections were not excluded.
- Communication was though normal department mass communication channels including intranet, bulletins, and mass distribution of posters and brochures. Coverage was spotty. An evaluation of the project revealed that some staff had never heard of the program.
- The project was implemented despite the delay in the infrastructure roll-out, so that staff were offered the opportunity to learn how to use the tools before the means to apply them was available.
- The narrow bandwidth and limited infrastructure disadvantaged rural health professionals. Many rural health professionals were not able to access the network. The first modules were eventually offered in print.
- Although endorsed by senior management, the program met with limited response. Four hundred computing skills packages were distributed in the first three weeks of their release. Interest in other modules was lower.

The project officially operated for two years.

Telehealth Project

Objectives were to establish a region-wide telehealth system to:

- enhance the access to health services for rural and remote communities and individuals in the region
- contribute to improved community-based health care
- improve the health status of rural and remote communities in the region.

The three-year project proposed to develop a hub-and-spoke model of services, connecting the three large regional hospitals to rural and remote locations across the region. Phase one was to assess the viability and cost effectiveness of telehealth for a range of uses, including clinical service delivery, peer support, education, and administration.

The system was expected to help reduce the isolation of rural and remote health professionals by offering a means for support and professional development. It also represented a significant change to the method of service delivery for rural and remote communities, where patients often travelled long distances for specialist consultations. The system also required changes from specialist clinicians as they were often required to move to a dedicated videoconference room to conduct a consultation with the patient and primary care provider.

Box 10.4 describes the management structures and processes of the project.

BOX 10.4 TELEHEALTH PROJECT MANAGEMENT PROCESS

- A Clinical Reference and Management Group was established to advise on key clinical and service delivery issues. This group included representatives from sections, the project team, and senior department management.
- Ongoing consultations with key players were enabled through the establishment of a Project Steering Committee.
- The project required the support of Rural and Community Health and Hospitals Services sections.
- The project sponsor was the manager of Rural and Community Health section. He understood the potential impact of the telehealth systems, stating that the project presented a new paradigm for service delivery.
- The project manager and team were located within Rural and Community Health and were responsible to the manager of that section. The project manager had limited authority, particularly in Hospitals Services.
- The managers of Hospitals Services were concerned that the project should not be an additional drain on resources, nor alter current referral patterns to the large regional hospitals in any significant way.
- A major challenge was addressing issues relating to appropriate hardware, software, and reliable telecommunications connections.
- A strategic decision was made to consciously adopt a people and service delivery (socio-technical) focus, rather than a technology focus. This included involving local communities and identifying telehealth 'champions' within each. This set the foundations for the project's future sustainability.
- The project team adopted a formal change model.
- Training focused primarily on the use of the technology and did not consider the changes in roles and relationships the use of the systems would necessarily bring.
- Inhibiting factors included issues around confidentiality, duty of care, and reimbursement.

The project began when telehealth was in its infancy. It was a complex project with multiple stakeholders, internal and external dependencies, and risks. In the first two years, six spoke sites and three hub sites were established. Use of the systems was initially slow, due to high call costs, unreliable quality of transmissions, and difficulty using the software. The major users were mental health services and diabetes support and education. Almost half of the calls made were for professional development and education.

Today, with twenty-seven sites across the region, telehealth has become an established tool for the delivery of services to rural and remote communities. Professional collaboration and education are the major uses, while clinical consultations are relatively low. The system uses a mix of broadband and high-speed secure digital telephone lines.

Community client management system

This system is currently in the planning stage. The aim is to replace the current paper-based system, which limits information sharing, with a regional electronic record system. It will be a Web-based application, featuring:

- standard electronic templates and workflows
- compliance with multiple National Minimum Dataset
- compliance with national and state reporting requirements utilising automated facilities
- internal and external information exchange
- procedures to identify and process reimbursable clients
- mobile computing facilities for data capture at point of care
- strategies to progress the interface between this system and the region's Hospital Information Systems.

This project will need to resolve structure, messaging, and security issues.

ANALYSIS

The description of this regional health department, and the projects it implemented, demonstrates a number of points discussed in this book. These include:

- The organisation exhibits the complex hierarchical structure typical of health organisations. The dominant culture reflects the influence of the biomedical health professions. At the same time, some sections also exhibit the flatter management structures that have been emerging, with the trend towards community-based, interdisciplinary care.
- Professional subcultures are evident, creating some conflict and rivalry between the two sections across which the systems operate.
- The organisation adopted the typical project-based approach to health informatics programs.

- At the time the projects were introduced, the organisation demonstrated an ad hoc, piecemeal approach to IT, with an emphasis on desktop technology, rather than a commitment to the development of regional infrastructure.
- The lack of strategic IT planning meant that the organisation had the typical silo arrangement of hardware, software, and network technology.

These characteristics are not atypical and therefore the challenges, successes, and failures will be applicable to many health organisations. The critical success factors discussed in Chapter 6 provide a framework for exploring how these characteristics impacted on the management of the projects.

Technical issues surrounding the introduction and implementation of health informatics systems into health care environments are well documented elsewhere. This analysis will focus on cultural and organisational issues since the key to organisational success for health informatics is the involvement of people in the assessment and design of systems. This helps to ensure that their needs are considered and addressed and that their interfaces are customised with the systems they use in their daily work.

The analysis of critical success factors demonstrates the socio-technical perspective adopted by both projects. This enabled the managers and teams to deal with a number of the cultural and organisation factors.

Critical success factors (CSFs) in action

A federal approach

As was discussed in Chapter 6, information resources should support the broad critical functions of the organisation, and new systems need to be considered in the context of the organisation's strategic goals and direction. This facilitates their eventual integration into an enterprise-wide system. The projects implemented by the regional health organisation might appear to be part of an overall strategic plan, with the infrastructure roll-out and the education program supporting the introduction of a telehealth network introduced to meet the organisation's goal of maintaining or enhancing health services in rural and remote areas. That this is not so is indicated by both the rapid change of emphasis from systems to support health care delivery to financial management systems, and the lack of any links, either in documentation or management structures, between the projects. Rather than considering the wider organisation context, each project reflected the typical silo mentality and focusing on immediate issues or on the interests of project sponsors.

Health informatics project

The lack of strategic integration clearly impacted on this project as the delayed infrastructure roll-out severely limited its capacity to deliver. More significantly, the primary reason for the project disappeared and the program was thus offered in a vacuum.

Telehealth project

The telehealth project supported the organisation's goals of maintaining health care services to rural and remote areas. The implementation of the grogram, however, reflected the traditional silo approach. For example, there was an opportunity for the telehealth project to draw on the education program to complement training. Telehealth project resources allowed for limited training, and this focused on skill development. The health informatics education program adopted a broader focus that would have dealt with issues around the cultural and organisational impacts of the technology, which are fundamental to the success of many projects.

Management support

In a large organisation, support of the most senior management will facilitate the availability of required resources for the project. The support of section and subsection managers will ensure projects are implemented. Executive level support was instrumental in establishing both projects. Varying levels of support from other levels of management impacted on the implementation of each project.

Health informatics project

There appeared to be a discrepancy between documented support and actions that assisted staff to readily participate in the program. Pressure to contain costs saw management reluctant to provide the resources to enable staff to participate. The majority of participants reported that, rather than being able to use workplace computers, they accessed the materials from their home computer. Evaluation of the project suggests that without active management support, many staff were unwilling to make a commitment beyond their normal work responsibilities. Where management actively supported the project, participation was high. Box 10.5 illustrates this.

BOX 10.5 MANAGEMENT SUPPORT

One manager of a district nursing service negotiated with the department to lease six computers, which were located in the district offices. Staff were given two hours per week to work through the materials. Most staff completed several modules.

The manager of a rural and remote home care program organised four workshops of three hours each, which staff were expected to attend. At the completion of the workshops, all participating staff had the skills to use basic software applications in their everyday work activities. This included using the Internet to find out information on client conditions.

Telehealth project

Management support for the telehealth program varied between the two sections. Support from the Rural and Community Health section was strong, since it was known that the manager was the project sponsor. The project team was able to involve key stakeholders in rural and remote facilities in consultations, demonstrations, and trials and this facilitated acceptance of telehealth. Managers in Hospitals & Ambulance expressed some reservations about resources and increased work loads. Support within this division ranged from guarded support to outright hostility. The location of project staff may have influenced management support. One team member was physically located within a hospital, while the rest were located within general administrative areas of the department, possibly contributing to the perception that telehealth was not an integral part of Hospitals & Ambulance.

Project champion

While a project champion is a critical success factor, the location of that individual within the organisation will impact on the extent of his or her influence. While a champion at senior management level is desirable, a clinician will be particularly beneficial where the project has a clinical focus. In both projects initiated by the regional health service, a champion with influence across the sections and professions would have been an advantage.

Health informatics project

A project sponsor initiated the education project, but restructuring of the department saw that individual disappear in the time between formal approval of the project and establishment of the project team. Since the project was managed and implemented externally, there was no champion within the organisation.

Telehealth project

The manager of Rural and Community Health was the project sponsor. He strongly supported telehealth within that section. He was, however, able to exert little influence on the Hospital Services section, which viewed the project with suspicion. The telehealth team actively pursued the identification and support of champions, particularly in the rural sites, and this proved to be one of the key success factors of this project.

Project management

Project managers of both programs did not have the authority to require staff to participate in programs or use the systems. They were thus dependent on persuasion to convince health professionals of the benefits of the projects.

Health informatics project

The project manager was located outside the health department and had no authority to require staff to participate. He therefore needed to find a means to persuade them to enrol in the program. This was difficult. While visionary, the offering of health informatics education before it could be applied resulted in many health professionals seeing the program as irrelevant. Lack of any formal recognition for completion of the modules compounded the issue.

Telehealth project

The need to work across two sections with very different management structures was challenging. Although the project team adopted a formal management process with relevant planning documentation and governance, their day-to-day management approach was much more informal, with few written records. Champions were recruited and contacts made through personal approaches. This reflected the structural, cultural, and management characteristics of Rural and Community Health, which worked well in that division. It worked less well in Hospitals Services, as seen in Box 10.6, where the team fell foul of the complex, multiple management structures discussed in Chapter 1.

BOX 10.6

FALLING FOUL OF COMPLEX MANAGEMENT STRUCTURES

The project team had negotiated a teleradiology project directly with the clinicians involved. Senior administrators of the hospitals were concerned had not been consulted. The administrators refused to pay the associated costs of the project. This particular project was never instituted.

Inadvertently crossing areas of authority and responsibility affected the program. This points to the difficulties around identifying an appropriate methodology for a complex organisation.

Project team membership

As noted in Chapter 6, project team members should be drawn from both the IT/IS area and the various departments and professional groups who will be using the programs or systems. The importance of this is demonstrated in the two projects.

Health informatics project

The project was planned and implemented by the project manager alone. The project advisory committee included representatives from the training institution and the health organisation. This was not representative of the health organisation and may have contributed to the difficulties experienced in disseminating information, generating management support, and involving staff in the project.

Telehealth project

The management team was specifically employed for the project. However, the several advisory committees ensured that a wide cross-section of views was able to be heard.

End-user input and participation

The consequences of limited end-user involvement are seen in both projects.

Health informatics project

The breadth of the project precluded extensive consultation. Needs analyses, surveys, and other data did enable end-user needs to be met to a certain extent, as is indicated by an analysis of survey responses leading to decisions to move from a wholly online program to one consisting of a combination of print-based and electronic, and to introduce basic computing skills as the first module.

Telehealth project

The nature of the project enabled extensive end-user consultations. There appeared to be some gaps in the process as indicated in the project evaluation, where issues around the adequacy of training, location of the equipment, and demands on staff time were raised.

Change management

The telehealth management team adopted a planned approach to change management, while the health informatics education program relied on the diffusion process.

Health informatics project

The health informatics education program adopted a diffusion model, which depended on potential participants hearing about and seeing the materials used to facilitate a more effective, easier way to work. The slow-down of the infrastructure roll-out resulted in health informatics education being offered in a vacuum, with no clearly perceived reason to participate. The complexity of the organisation also appeared to impact on successful diffusion. Organisation characteristics thought to facilitate diffusion include size, degree of centralisation of power and control, complexity of professional groups, the relative emphasis on rules and procedures, availability of uncommitted resources, and voluntary or involuntary adoption. Overall, the regional health system was formal and centralised. However, the size and complexity of the organisation meant that these characteristics varied widely across the divisions. Current thinking suggests an innovation may be successfully introduced into most environments if the particular characteristics of an organisation, or sections of an organisation, are matched with strategies to introduce the innovation. An external manager who is not familiar with the complexities of the organisation would have some difficulty in doing so.

Telehealth project

Once again, the need to work across two quite different sections required a systematic approach to change management. The formal model adopted by the telehealth team, which involved the development of extensive documentation in terms of plans, timelines, resource needs, task lists, risk analyses, and evaluation procedures, was standard procedure for the organisation. This was a somewhat cumbersome process but ensured that coordination and control were maintained in a complex project. The team supplemented these formal processes with extensive stakeholder consultation, recruit-ment of local champions, and informal networking. This worked very effectively in the spoke sites, but not so effectively in the complex hierarchies of the hospital hub sites.

Communication

The different approaches adopted by each project impacted on their ability to com-municate effectively with significant groups.

Health informatics project

Given the breadth of the target group, communication was via the mass communica-tion channels of the department. This proved to be somewhat unpredictable. Not all staff had access to the intranet and the distribution of brochures and newsletters was dependent on managers of each section and subsection. A rash of enquiries from a particular ward, section, or centre indicated that materials had been distributed. The erratic coverage undoubtedly impacted on the project.

Telehealth project

From the beginning, the project team demonstrated an awareness of the need to mar-ket the technology, and the opportunities inherent within it, to various stakeholders. For rural sites, a strategy was developed that targeted key groups prior to the estab-lishment of any telehealth facility, extensive consultations were held to gauge interest and establish local management groups. Services were negotiated prior to connection to each new site. The management team were very aware of the need for sites to be involved and to have some ownership of the project. This was particularly the case in hub sites. In the past, specialist clinicians had not been required to travel. Patients came to them. For some specialists, face-to-face consultations were preferable. The quality of transmissions made telehealth unsuitable for dermatology, for example. Thus, there was no immediate, obvious benefit, but instead a potential for increased demands for already stretched services.

The telehealth team did appear to neglect connectivity and interface issues, which impacted on user expectations. Calls using the first systems were expensive, leading many users to opt for the lowest-speed transmissions. These were often poor quality and unsuitable for many consults. In addition, the software was difficult to navigate, result-ing in frequent disconnections. Evaluation of the first phase of the project found wide-spread user dissatisfaction with connectivity and user-interface aspects of the project.

End-user skill development

The health informatics project was about skill development, while the telehealth man-agement team viewed skill development as an integral part of the project.

Health informatics project

The project was intended to develop the skills and knowledge to enable health profes-sionals to use the health informatics systems. Significant resources were expended and a training organisation was given responsibility for developing the materials. The com-plexity of the health department meant that the materials needed to cater for a range of skill levels and capacity to access appropriate technology. Usability was emphasised, particularly in those modules introducing participants to online learning. The response from participants suggests that skill development was successful although limited.

Telehealth project

The telehealth project conducted a series of skill development workshops. These were voluntary and informal. While this introduced staff to the technology, participant evaluations expressed concerns that there was insufficient hands-on experience or practice time. Since the telehealth connections made during training had to be paid for, ensuring adequate practice was a challenge. It was, however, significant for the project as the usability of applications was low. A consistent criticism during the evaluation of the first phase of the project was the difficulty of using the technology. The training focused on skills and did not address the issue of changes to work routines and work processes. Given that telehealth does change roles, relationships, and routines, lack of attention to this issue in the training was a significant oversight.

This discussion has explored the way a health organisation sought to apply health informatics to resolve some of the day-to-day issues of health care delivery to rural and remote areas. The potential to use health informatics at a strategic level might also be considered.

Strategic health informatics

While many of the challenges for rural health, including the issues of timely access to specialist medical and other health services and access to information, education, and training opportunities, are being tackled through the use of information and communications systems, a real opportunity for health informatics to make a difference in the delivery of rural and remote care lies in its potential for strategic information management. Automation of information systems allows more effective integration of data and information, which can be used to support information management and decision-making activities in policy and planning, patient care, education, and research in order to meet some of the challenges currently confronting rural health. Health data and information, aggregated by combining many sets of individual records stored in complex health databases, can be analysed and interpreted to inform regional and national health policy and planning purposes.

Health informatics applications afford the opportunity to reframe rural health priorities, which are based on sound evidence and research through merging data on health status, community priority setting, provider priority setting, and partner priority setting within a research framework.

SUMMARY

This chapter brought together a number of key aspects of earlier chapters by looking at the applications of health informatics in the context of rural health.

One of the major challenges for rural and remote communities was explored: access to health and related services. This began by recognising the diversity and heterogeneity of rural and remote communities and the similar differentiation of health status in these communities. Data does suggest, however, that health status progressively worsens as population density and infrastructure decreases. The difficulties of timely access to health and related services underpin the health differentials between urban and rural populations.

Many of the challenges facing rural health are being addressed through a health informatics approach but an understanding of all the facets of the tools of health informatics is important for sustainability and success. The issues that confront urban services include technical and security standards, usability, and professional and cultural aspects. The case study of a how a regional health service utilised a health informatics approach to rural health illustrated how these factors impact on the success of health informatics systems.

The chapter concluded by suggesting that health informatics has much potential at a strategic level with the collection and analysis of health data facilitated by integrated health information systems being used to inform policy and strategy at state and national levels.

WWW LINKS

National Rural Health Alliance Inc. (Australia) <http://www.ruralhealth.org.au>

Health Canada, Rural Health <http://www.hc-sc.gc.ca/english/ruralhealth/>

Rural health in New Zealand and Australia: *Health Care and Informatics Review Online*
<http://www.enigma.co.nz/hcro/website/index.cfm?fuseaction=archiveissue&issueid=28>

AMA position statement on rural and remote health <http://www.ama.com.au/web.nsf/doc/SHED-5FY79F>

Health Canada: Health infostructure in Canada, provincial and territorial plans and priorities <http://www.hc-sc.gc.ca/ohih-bsi/chics/pt/yt_e.html>

CRITICAL THINKING

A small rural community has been invited to participate in a project to trial several information and communications systems applications for the delivery of health care services.

1 Identify applications that could be included in such a trial and explain how they might resolve some of the problems of providing health care to rural and remote communities.

2 Discuss the advantages and drawbacks of the proposed project from the perspective of key stakeholders.

3 How valid is the view that information and communications systems are a means of reducing face-to-face services to rural and remote communities?

4 What steps would you take to ensure the successful introduction of a health informatics application to a rural and remote community?

5 How would you measure 'successful introduction'?

Glossary

andragogy
The practice of teaching adults, based on assumptions that adults need reasons for learning, need to learn by experience, approach learning as problem solving, and learn best when the topic is of immediate value.

behaviourism
Psychological learning theories that explain learning in terms of conditioning. Stimulus–response theory, pioneered by Ivan Pavlov, is one of the earliest behaviourist theories.

biomedicine
Application of scientific principles of biology and physiology to the understanding and treatment of disease.

bureaucracy
A way of structuring human organisations based on rational decision-making.

clinical decision support system (CDSS)
An information system designed to assist the health professional with clinical decision-making.

cognitive learning theories
Theories that seek to explain how information is taken into the brain, how it is processed, in what form it is exhibited by the learner, and how behaviour can be altered by feedback.

cognitive overload
A condition occurring as the result of excessive demands made on the cognitive processes, particularly memory.

concept
A word or phrase that encapsulates an idea, object, or process.

confidentiality
The requirement that information will only be used for the purpose for which it was gathered.

culture
The values, beliefs, assumptions, and behaviours that shape the behaviour of a society, community, or other organised group of people.

data

Raw, unanalysed facts. A simple example is the numbers 39.5, 37.5, and 38.5. These numbers have no context or meaning.

differentiation

As scientific knowledge increases, it divides, or differentiates into different disciplines and sub-disciplines.

diffusion

The process of communicating information about a new process or idea to members of an organisation or other social system.

diffusion of innovation

A theory used to explain the patterns of adoption of new products or processes. It is used frequently to explain the adoption of technology.

diseases of affluence

Diseases that are attributed to affluent Western lifestyles. They include cancer, heart disease, stroke, diabetes, and lung disease.

e-health

The use of information and communication technology to deliver health services. This includes services and activities conducted within the parameters of established health systems and services, and activities available in the broader community, most frequently via the Internet.

empirical knowledge

Knowledge obtained through the senses.

evidence-based practice

The practice of acquiring, analysing, and applying current best evidence when making decisions about the care of individual patients.

expert system

An information system that assists with decisions by organising facts and knowledge—which are stored in a database—into rules that are applied to a given set of questions or symptoms.

explicit knowledge

Formal, structured knowledge. It can be expressed verbally or in print and transmitted to others. It is easy to share through such mechanisms as formulae, protocols, care pathways, rules, and databases.

fuzzy knowledge

Knowledge that is incomplete or imprecise, and where interpretation is a matter of degree.

globalisation

An ongoing process of increasing integration of the popular, or mass culture political integration in the form of international trade and the growing influence of transnational corporations.

Health*Connect*

An electronic health records network being developed by the Australian Government.

health consumer
A term being used to convey that 'patients' are being increasingly considered as equal partners, capable of making choices and decisions with regard to their own health and medical care.

health informatics
An emerging scientific discipline that adopts a socio-technical approach to the collection, storage, analysis, and communication of health-related data, information, and knowledge.

health information system (HIS)
An automated or manual system that includes people, machines, and processes for gathering, storing, and processing health data, and communicating health information to users at the right time and in the right place.

humanism
An approach to learning that argues that people are in a process of constant personal growth, that they naturally want to learn, and are best able to decide for themselves what and how they should learn.

hypothesis
A measurable (testable) statement that the researcher seeks to prove in the course of the research.

individual knowledge
Individual knowledge resides within individuals and is manifested through individual skills or expertise.

informatics
Science focusing on the use of information technology for the storing and processing of data.

information
Data that is interpreted, organised, or structured in a meaningful way.

information society
A term used to indicate the increasing importance of information in contemporary society. Information has become a valuable resource, and is generating wealth for individuals, companies, and countries in the same way that manufacturing did in the last century.

innovation
An idea, practice, or object that is perceived as new by the individuals or organisation to which it is introduced. Potential users compare the innovation to existing ideas, practices, and objects before making a decision about whether to adopt the innovation or not.

jargon
Specialised terminology or concepts for a particular area or discipline.

knowledge
The capacity to make sense of and use data and information.

knowledge management
Seeks to make implicit information explicit.

legacy system

An information system that runs on obsolete hardware, is expensive and difficult to maintain, and almost impossible to expand or integrate with other systems.

MEDLARS

A medical information database developed by the US National Library of Medicine during the 1960s. MEDLARS stands for Medical Literature Analysis and Retrieval System.

Medline

A large database of abstracts of articles in the international medical journals at the US National Library of Medicine.

MedlinePlus

A large database of health-related information for consumers. It is a service provided by the US National Library of Medicine and the National Institutes of Health.

messaging standards

Establish a format and a sequence for data transmission to enable sharing of health information. A medical message, for example, might require the first segment of a message to identify the sending and receiving systems, the type of message and the name, date of birth, and unique identifier of the individual who is the subject of the message.

model

A small copy or representation of an object, abstract process, or planned entity or process.

MYCIN

An expert system developed during the 1970s for diagnosing and recommending treatment for bacterial infections of the blood.

norms

A rules or guideline for acceptable behaviour. Norms can be formal, such as protocols for dispensing drugs, or informal, such as ways of addressing particular groups of staff.

organisation

A group of people organised into a stable, structured relationship of clearly defined roles and responsibilities, working together to achieve a common goal.

organisational climate

The climate is the 'atmosphere' of the workplace. An organisation may have a climate that encourages tradition and routine, or it may have a climate that supports experimentation and trying new ways of working. The climate is how you 'feel' about your work environment.

organisational knowledge

Knowledge required to perform business operations or make effective decisions. Individual knowledge contributes to the pool of organisational knowledge. Therefore, organisational knowledge may be viewed as collective knowledge.

personally identifiable data (PID)
Data that can uniquely identify an individual.

personally identified information (PII)
Information that can uniquely identify an individual.

positivist research
An approach to social research modelled on the physical sciences. It stresses evidence acquired through the senses.

power
The ability to achieve your aims or further your own interests, even when others disagree or oppose you.

privacy
Refers to the right of an individual to limit access by others to personal information.

product attributes
Characteristics of software such as screen layout, menus, and consistency, which impact on the usability of the product.

profession
An occupation requiring specialised knowledge and skills.

rapid applications development (RAD)
An approach to systems development that is inherently designed to provide fast development with better quality results than the traditional waterfall approach.

role
A set of expectations that define how the person occupying a particular status or position should act.

security
Protection of data and information. There are three dimensions of information protection: access, integrity, and availability.

security standards
Designed to protect data from unauthorised or inadvertent access to, or disclosure of, information.

silo system
An information system, often a legacy system, serving a department or a purpose, independent of other information systems in the enterprise.

socio-technical
A perspective that seeks to understand the dynamics between technology and the social environment in which it is used.

standard
Widely accepted rules or specifications that enable health professionals to collect, store, and share health-related data, information, and knowledge in an electronic format.

status
A sociological concept used to describe a position in a social structure. Is also used as a measure of social prestige or social standing.

structure and content standards
Used to provide descriptions of the data elements to be included in documents to be shared.

subculture
Variations or adaptations of the values, beliefs, assumptions, and behaviours that comprise the culture of the organisation.

systems theory
A theory that studies an entity, such as a health organisation, as a system of interacting parts.

tacit knowledge
Derives from personal experience and can involve subjective insight, intelligence, and intuition. It resides in people's minds.

technocentric
The tendency to focus on technology and technological issues, rather than viewing technology as part of a wider system that enables a focus on both technical and non-technical issues.

theory
The foundation of a discipline. Theories are used to explain what the physical or social world is like, how that world changes, and why it changes.

usability
Refers to software attributes including ease of learning, efficiency and effectiveness of use, error minimisation, and the feeling of satisfaction experienced by the user.

user orientation
Used in the context of software usability, and includes previous experience with technology, professional role, and the nature of the tasks the user may be required to perform.

user performance
Focuses on how well the software enables users to successfully fulfil their work tasks.

vocabularies
Concerned with developing standard terminology to describe symptoms, diagnoses, treatments, and care.

workflow
Tasks or procedures broken into a number of steps, with each step being performed by a different individual.

work routine
Routines are repetitive patterns of behaviour that structure our activities and interactions. Health professionals develop routines to enable them to more efficiently complete their daily tasks. They can be informal habits, such as personal routine, or formal and explicit, such as hospital protocols for screening newborn infants.

worldview
Ideas and assumptions that shape the way we view and understand the world.

Bibliography

Abbott, P. 2002, 'Introducing nursing informatics', *Nursing*, January, vol. 32, no. 1, p. 14.

Advisory Council on Health Infostructure 2001, 'Toward electronic health records', Office of Health and the Information Highway, Health Canada, Ottawa, <http://www.hc-sc.gc.ca/ohih-bsi/pubs/2001_ehr_dse/ehr_dse_e.html>, viewed 10 December 2004.

Alberta Government 2003, 'New electronic health record launched', <http://www.gov.ab.ca/home/index.cfm?Page=580>, viewed 15 December 2004.

Alter, S.L. 1980, *Decision Support Systems: Current Practices and Continuing Challenges*, Addison-Wesley, Reading, MA.

Altman, R. 1997, 'Informatics in the care of patients: ten notable challenges', *Western Journal of Medicine*, vol. 166, no. 2, pp. 118–22.

Alvarez C. 2002. *The promise of e-health—a Canadian perspective*, Internet Health <http://www. virtualmed.netfirms.com/internethealth/ehi200214.html>, viewed November 2004.

American National Standards Institute 2004, 'New standards, products and services', <http://webstore.ansi.org/ansidocstore/default.asp?> viewed 14 October 2004.

American Nurses Association 1995, 'Position paper on computer-based patient records standards', <http://nursingworld.org/readroom/position/joint/jtcpri1.htm>, viewed 1 November 2004.

Anderson, J. 1997, 'Clearing the way for physicians' use of clinical information systems', *Communications of the ACM*, August, vol. 40, no. 8, p. 83.

Anogianakis, G., Ilonidis, G., Anogeianaki, A., Milliaras, S., Klisarova, A., Temelkov, T. & Vlachakis-Milliaras, E. 2003, 'Developing prison telemedicine systems: the Greek experience', *Journal of Telemedicine and Telecare*, vol. 9, supplement 2, pp. 2–4.

Annan, K. 2003, 'Address to the World Summit on the information society', WSIS, Geneva, <http://www.itu.int/wsis/geneva/coverage/statements/opening/annan.html>, viewed 4 October 2004.

Arocha, J. 2003, 'What is health informatics?', Department of Health Studies and Gerontology, University of Waterloo, Ontario.

Atkinson, C., Tillal, E., Paul, R., & Pouloudi, A. 2001, 'Investigating integrated socio-technical approaches to health informatics', *34th Hawaii International Conference on System Sciences*, 3–6 January 2001.

Australian Bureau of Statistics 2002, *Australian Social Trends 1999, Population—Population Trends: Our Aging Population*, ABS, Canberra <http://www.abs.gov.au/Ausstats/abs@.nsf/0/b7760619c3973594ca25699f0005d60f?OpenDocument>, viewed 20 October 2004.

Australian Health Ministers Advisory Council (AHMAC) 2003, *Healthy Horizons: Outlook 2003 – 2007*, a joint development of AHMAC's National Rural Health Policy Sub-committee and the National Rural Health Alliance, Canberra.

Bashshur, R. & Shannon, G.R. 2002, 'The evolution of telemedicine/telehealth technology and the Internet', SymbiosisOnline.com, August, <http://symbiosisonline.com/aug02_telemedic.htm>, viewed 2 February 2003.

Beaumont, R. 1999, 'Types of health information systems', <http://www.robin-beaumont.co.uk/rbeaumont/virtualclassroom/chap12/s2/systems1.htm>, viewed 23 September 2004.

Beginners Central 1998, 'A users guide to the Internet', Northern Webs, Sagle, ID, <http://www.northernwebs. com/bc/> viewed 23 September 2004.

Begley, R.J., Riege, M., Rosenblum, J. & Tseng, D. 2000, 'Adding Intelligence to Medical Devices', <http://www.devicelink.com/mddi/archive/00/03/014.html>, viewed 13 October 2004.

Bentivoglio, J. 2003, 'Unleash the Internet', Professional Plus Inc., <http://www.profplus.com/article052001.php>, viewed 9 August 2004.

Berwick, D.M. 2002, 'Escape fire: lessons for the future of health care', The Commonwealth Fund, New York, <http://www.members.cox.net/trustmemedblog/escapefire.pdf>, viewed 1 October 2004.

Bilton, T., Bonnett, K., Jones, P., Skinner, D., Stanworth, M. & Webster, A. 1996, *Introductory Sociology*, 3rd edn, Macmillan, London.

Bouchier, H. & Bath, P.A. 2003, 'Evaluation of websites that provide information on Alzheimer's disease', *Health Informatics Journal*, vol. 9, no. 1, pp. 17–31.

Bowns, R., Rotherham, G. & Paisley, S. 1999, 'Factors associated with success in the implementation of information management and technology in the NHS', *Health Informatics Journal*, vol. 5, pp. 136–45.

Briggs, B. 2001, 'Doctors sound off on IT concerns', *Health Data Management*, New York, vol. 9, no. 1, pp. 38–48.

Briggs, B. 2005, 'Will electronic records become routine?', *Health Data Management*, vol. 9, no. 1, pp. 38–48.

Brown, N. 1995, 'A brief history of telemedicine', Telemedicine Information Exchange, <http://tie.telemed.org/telemed101/understand/tm_history.asp>, viewed 22 November 2003.

Carlson, B. 1996, 'Technology offers an answer to information overload', *Managed Care Magazine*, <http://www.managedcaremag.com/archives/9612/MC9612.clinicalsoft.shtml>, viewed 11 June 2004.

Carter, M. 2000, 'Integrated electronic health records and patient privacy: possible benefits but real dangers: strategies to develop integrated electronic health records must address consumer concerns, not dismiss them with claims of the public good', *Medical Journal of Australia*, vol. 172, no. 1, pp. 28–30.

Celler B.G. & Lovell, N.H. 2003, 'Home telecare for the management', CD ROM, vol. 1, HIC 2003 RACGP Combined Conferences, Sydney, 10–12 August.

Chew, M., & Van Der Weyden, M. 2002, 'Surveying the specialist silos', *Medical Journal of Australia*, vol. 176, no. 1, p. 2 <http://www.mja.com.au/public/issues/176_01_070102/ che10824_0fm.html>, viewed 23 March 2004.

Children's Hospital at Westmead 2003, 'Look, no paper!', Public Relations Department, <http://www.chw.edu.au/about/news/items/paperless_medical_records.htm>, viewed 22 September 2004.

Clarke, R. 2001, 'Research challenges in emergent e-health technologies', <http://www.anu.edu.au/people/Roger.Clarke/EC/eHlthRes.html#Ben>, viewed 12 September 2004.

Coiera, E. 1997, *Guide to Medical Informatics, the Internet and Telemedicine*, Arnold, London.

Coiera, E. 2003, *Guide to Health Informatics*, Arnold, London.

Coiera, E. 2004, 'Four rules for the reinvention of health care', *British Medical Journal*, vol. 328 no. 7449 pp. 1197–9, <http://bmj.bmjjournals.com/cgi/content/full/326/7449/1197>, viewed 13 June 2004.

Coffield, F. (ed.) 2000, *Differing Visions of the Learning Society, Research Findings*, vols I and II, Policy Press, Bristol.

Commonwealth Fund 2003, International Survey of Hospital Executives, Commonwealth Fund Harvard/Harris Intereactive, <http://www.cmwf.org/usr_doc/2003_IHP_Survey_Chartpack.pdf> viewed October 2004.

Cornford, T. & Klecun-Dabrowska, E. 2003, 'Images of health technology in national and local strategies', *Methods of Information in Medicine*, vol. 42, no. 4, pp. 353–9.

Darbyshire, P. 2004, '"Rage against the machine?": nurses' and midwives' experiences of using computerized information systems for clinical information', *Journal of Clinical Nursing*, vol. 13, pp. 17–25.

Degeling, P., Maxwell, S., Kennedy, J. & Coyle, B. 2003, 'Medicine, management, and modernisation: a "danse macabre"?', *British Medical Journal*, 326, pp. 649–52.

Delucca, J. & Enmark, R. 2000, 'E-Health: the changing model of healthcare', *Frontiers of Health Service Management*, Fall, vol. 17, no. 1, pp. 3–15.

Department of Health and Ageing, Australia 2002, *National Health Priorities and Quality*, Department of Health and Ageing Publications, Canberra <http://www.health.gov.au/internet/wcms/publishing.nsf/Content/Health+ Priorities-1>, viewed 3 March 2004.

Department of Health and Ageing, Australia 2004, *Health Fact Sheet 5—A Health System Evolving through Technology*, <http://www.health.gov.au/internet/wcms/Publishing.nfs/Content/health-budget2004-h>, viewed 14 August 2004.

Department of Health and Family Services 1998, Developing an Active Australia: a framework for physical activity and health, Department of Health and Family Services, Canberra, <http://health.gov.au/internet/wcms/Publishing.nsf/Content/health-pubhlth-publicat-document-active-cnt.htm>, viewed October 2004.

Dillon, E. & Loermans, J. 2003, 'Telehealth in Western Australia: the challenge of evaluation', *Journal of Telemedicine and Telecare*, vol. 9, supplement 2, pp. 15–19.

Duffett-Leger, L. 1996, 'Looking to the future: nursing and entrepreneurship nursing: change, challenge, choice', Canadian Nursing Students' Association, <http://www.cnsa. ca/publications/connection/1996april/article10.php>, viewed 30 September 2004.

Engelbardt, S. & Nelson, R. 2002, *Health Care Informatics: An Interdisciplinary Approach*, Mosby Inc., St Louis, MO.

Ferguson, T. & Frydman, G. 2004, 'The first generation of e-patients', editorial, *British Medical Journal*, 328, pp. 1148–9, <http://bmj.bmjjournals.com/cgi/contentfull/328/7449/1146>, viewed 19 May 2004.

Fleet, M. 1998, 'Misspelling a factor in meningitis girl's death', *Electronic Telegraph*, <http://www.telegraph.co.uk/htmlContent.jhtml?html=/Farchive/1998/08/28/nmen28.html>, viewed 13 December 2004.

Forbes, T., Hallier, J. & Kelly, L. 2004, 'Doctors as managers: investors and reluctants in a dual role', *Health Services Management Research*, August, vol. 17, no. 3, pp. 167–77.

Fourman, M. 2002, 'Informatics', *Informatics Research Report*, EDI-INF-RR-0139, Chapter 2, University of Edinburgh, <http://www.inf.ed.ac.uk/publications/report/0139.html>, viewed 9 January 2004.

Gaillour, F. 1999, 'Rethinking the CPR: Is perfect the enemy of good', *Health Management Technology*, May, vol. 20, no. 4, pp. 22–6.

Gawande, A.A. & Bates, D.W. 2000, 'The use of information technology in improving medical performance', Parts II and III: Physician-Support Tools, *Medscape*, 14 and 22 February.

Gedda, R. 2004, 'NSW electronic health records system goes live', *CIO*, <http://www.cio.com.au/index.php/id;1113312711;fp;512;fpid;1435609079>, viewed 15 December 2004.

Georgiou, A. 2002, 'Data, information and knowledge: the health informatics model and its role in evidence-based medicine', *Journal of Evaluation in Clinical Practice*, vol. 8, no. 2, pp. 127–30.

Gillies, J. & Holt, A. 2003, 'Anxious about electronic health records? No need to be', *Journal of the New Zealand Medical Association*, 26 September, vol. 116, no. 1182, <http://www.nzma.org.nz/journal/116-1182/604/>, viewed 27 August 2004.

Glenn D. & Chung 2003, 'Go with the flow', *Health Management Technology*, vol. 24, no. 1, p. 66.

Gorry, G.A. & Scott-Morton, M.S. 1971, 'A framework for management information systems', *Sloan Management Review*, vol. 13, no. 1, pp. 55–71.

Greatbatch D., Murphy E. & Dingwall R. 2001, 'Evaluating medical information systems: ethnomethodological and interactionist approches', *Health Services Management Reseearch*, vol. 14, no. 3, pp 181–91.

Hailey, D. & Crowe, B. 2003, 'A profile of success and failure in telehealth—evidence and opinion from the success and failures in telehealth conferences', *Journal of Telemedicine and Telecare*, vol. 9, supplement 2, pp. 22–3.

Hannah, K., Ball, M. & Edwards, M. 1999, *Introduction to Nursing Informatics*, Springer-Verlag, New York.

Hannan, T., Tierney, W., Rotich, J., Smith, F., Bii, J., Einterz, R. & Mamlin, J. 2002, 'The Mosoriot Medical Record System, Eldoret, Kenya: capturing data to improve quality of care in sub-Saharan Africa', CD Rom, Proceedings, Tenth National Health Informatics Conference, 5–6 August, Melbourne.

Health Canada 2000, 'E-health: from vision to action', <http://www.hc-sc.gc.ca/ohih-bsi/pubs/newsbull/newsbull1_e.html>, viewed 9 July 2003.

Health Canada 2001, 'Toward Electronic Health Records', <http://www.hc-sc.gc.ca/ohih-bsi/pubs/2001_ehr_dse/ehr_dse_e.html>, viewed June 2004.

Health Canada 2002, 'Rural health/telehealth', The Health Transition Fund, Ottawa, <http://www.hc-sc.gc.ca/htf-fass/english/whatwedo_e.htm>, viewed 14 May 2004.

Health Canada 2004, E-health Resource Centre, Health and the Information Highway Division, Key Topics, <http://www.hc-sc.gc.ca/ohih-bsi/theme/index_e.html>, viewed 15 December 2004.

Health*Connect* 2004, 'Consent', <http://www.healthconnect.gov.au/building/Consent.htm>, viewed 17 July 2004.

Health Informatics Society of Australia (HISA), <http://www.hisa.org.au/default.php>, viewed 15 December 2004.

Health Level 7 (HL7) 2004, <http://www.hl7.org/>, viewed 10 January 2004.

Heathfield, H. & Wyatt, J. 1993, 'Philosophies for the design and development of clinical decision-support systems', *Methods of Information in Medicine*, vol. 32, no. 1, pp. 1–8.

Hersh, W.R. 2002, 'Medical informatics: improving health care through information', *Journal of the American Medical Association*, 23/30 October, vol. 288, no. 16, pp. 1955–8.

Heylighen, F. & Joslyn, C. 1992, 'What is systems theory?', Principia Cybernetica Web, <http://pespmc1.vub.ac.be/SYSTHEOR.html>, viewed 24 March 2004.

Horsfield, B. & Peterson, C. 2000, 'The hierarchy of discourses in the current diffusion of e-health, telemedicine and telehealth in Australia', Communications Research Forum, <http://www.crf.dcita.gov.au/papers2000/horsfield.doc>, viewed 15 December 2004.

Hunt, D., Haynes, R., Hanna, S. & Smith, K. 1998, 'Effects of computer-based clinical decision support systems on physician performance and patient outcomes: a systematic review', *Journal of the American Medical Association*, 21 October, vol. 280, no. 15, pp. 1339–46.

Jennet, P., Yeo, M., Pauls, M. & Graham, J. 2003, 'Organisational readiness for telemedicine: implications for success or failure', *Journal of Telemedicine and Telecare*, vol. 9, supplement 2, pp. 27–9.

Johns, M.L. 2002, *Information Management for Health Professions*, 2nd edn, Delmar (Thomson Learning), Albany, NY.

Kearsley, G. 2004, 'Explorations in Learning & Instruction: The Theory Into Practice Database', <http://tip.psychology.org> viewed August 2004.

Kelly, B. 2002, 'The future of card technology in health care', *Health Data Management*, May, vol. 10, no. 5, pp. 64–8.

Kerr, K. 2004, 'The electronic health record in New Zealand', *Healthcare and Informatics Review Online*, <http://www.enigma.co.nz/hcro/website/index.cfm?fuseaction=articledisplay&featureid=040304>, viewed 23 April 2004.

Kinyon, C. 2003, 'One CFO's success with transitioning to an automated patient record', *Healthcare Financial Management*, vol. 57, no. 2, pp. 52–6.

Klecun-Dabrowska, E. & Cornford, T. 2001, 'Evaluation and telehealth—an interpretive study', 34th Hawaii International Conference on System Sciences, 3–6 January.

KPMG Consulting 1999, 'Review of the literature on evaluation in telehealth', Commonwealth Department of Health and Aged Care and Australian and New Zealand Telehealth Committee.

Kropp, B. & Gallaher, M. 2001, 'Medical records vulnerable to ID theft', *Computer Security Digest*, vol. 19, no. 1, p. 3.

Lemieux-Charles, L., Meslin, E.M., Aird, C., Baker, R. & Leatt, P. 1993, 'Ethical issues faced by clinician/managers in resource-allocation', *Hospital and Health Services Administration*, Summer, vol. 38, no. 2, pp. 267.

Lewis, M. & Mitchell, J. 1998, *Electronic Patient Records: A Resource Manual*, Health Information Management Association of Australia, Sydney.

Lippman, H. 2000, 'Clinical decision support', *Hippocrates*, vol. 14, no. 3, <http://www.hippocrates.com/archive/March2000/03features/03cds.html>, viewed 20 March 2004.

Littlejohns P., Wyatt, C. & Garvican, L. 2003, 'Evaluating computerised health information systems: hard lessons still to be learnt', *British Medical Journal*, 19 April, 320, pp. 800–63.

Loue, S. & Quill, B. 2001, *Handbook of Rural Health*, Kluwer Academic/Plenum Publishers, New York.

Luciani, D., Marchesi, M. & Bertolini, G. 2003, 'The role of Bayesian Networks in the diagnosis of pulmonary embolism', *Journal of Thrombosis and Haemostasis*, vol. 1, pp. 698–707.

McAlearney, A., Schweikhart S. & Medow, M. 2004, 'Doctors' experience with handheld computers in clinical practice: qualitative study', *British Medical Journal*, vol. 328, no. 7449, p. 1162.

McCrosin, R. 2003, 'Managing risk in telemedicine', *Journal of Telemedicine and Telecare*, vol. 9, supplement 2, pp. 36–8.

McDonald, I., Hill, S., Daly, J. & Crowe, B. 1998, *Evaluating Telemedicine in Victoria: A Generic Framework*, Acute Health Division, Department of Human Services, Melbourne.

MacDougall, J. & Brittain, J. 1994, 'Health informatics', *Annual Review of Information Science and Technology*, vol. 29, Chapter 5, <http://www.asis.org/Publications/ARIST/arist-94/arist-94-section-3/arist-94-chapter5.html>, viewed 26 July 2004.

McGee, M. 2004, 'E-Health on the horizon', *Information Week*, 17 May, <http://www.informationweek.com/showArticle.jhtml?articleID=20300885>, viewed 30 May 2004.

McGill, A. 2001, 'The challenges for health informatics in Australia to 2005', Proceedings, HIC2001, Health Informatics Society of Australia, Canberra, 29–31 July.

McKenzie, B.C. 2000, 'What is health informatics?' <http://www.btinternet.com/~bioneural.net/health_informatics.html>, viewed 3 July 2003.

Maheu, M. 2000, 'Telehealth: delivering behavioural telehealth via the Internet (e-health)', *Telehealth Net*, <http://telehealth.net/articles/deliver.html>, viewed 11 February 2003.

Marakas, G.M. 2003, *Decision Support Systems in the 21st Century*, Prentice-Hall, Upper Saddle River, NJ.

Marckmann, G. 2001, 'Recommendations for the ethical development and use of medical decision-support systems', *Medscape Today*, <http://www.medscape.com/viewarticle/408143>, viewed 17 July 2004.

Marietti, C. 1998, 'Will the real CPR/EMR/EHR please stand up?' *Healthcare Informatics*, <http://www.healthcare-informatics.com/issues/1998/05_98/cover.htm>, viewed 19 November 2003.

Martin, E., Brown, C., DeHayes, D., Hoffer, J. & Perkins, W. 2002, *Managing Information Technology*, 4th edn, Prentice-Hall, NJ.

Milstein, R. 1999, 'Telemedicine—creating virtual certainty out of remote possibilities: an international, comparative analysis of policy, regulatory and medico-legal obstacles and solutions', Report for Department of Human Services (Victoria), abridged version, <http://www.dhs.vic.gov.au/ahs/archive/telemed/index.htm>, viewed 15 December, 2004.

Mitchell & Associates 1999, 'From telehealth to e-health: the unstoppable rise of e-health', Commonwealth Department of Communications, Information Technology and the Arts, <http://www.jma.com.au/ehealth_pubs.htm>, viewed 3 February 2003.

Moulton, D. 2004, 'Telehealth time-consuming but beneficial for N.S. MDs', *Medical Post*, vol. 40, no. 23, p. 47.

Musen, M.A. & van Bemmel, J.H. 2002, 'Challenges for medical informatics as an academic discipline: workshop report', *Yearbook of Medical Informatics*, International Medical Informatics Association and Schattauer GmbH, Stuttgart.

Musen, M.A. & van Bemmel, J.H. 2003, 'Challenges for medical informatics: a discipline coming of age', *Yearbook of Medical Informatics*, International Medical Informatics Association and Schattauer GmbH, Stuttgart.

National Centre for Policy Analysis 2000, 'Patient dissatisfaction', <http://www.ncpa.org/ba/ba311/ba311.html>, viewed 30 September 2004.

National Electronic Health Records Taskforce 2000, *A Health Information Network for Australia*, Commonwealth Department of Health and Aged Care, Canberra.

National Health Service Information Authority 2001, 'Professional qualifications for NHS health informatics specialists', <http://www.nhsia.nhs.uk/informatics/pages/resource_informatics/prof_qual.pdf>, viewed 27 February 2004.

National Health Service National Programme for Information Technology 2003, 'The public view on electronic health records', <http://www.dh.gov.uk/assetRoot/04/05/50/46/04055046.pdf>, viewed 15 December 2004.

National Institute of Clinical Studies 2004, Report on the Electronic Decision Support Governance Workshop, <http://www.nicsl.com.au/pdf/html/0.html>, viewed December 2004.

National Rural Health Alliance 2002, 'Healthy horizons: progress against the healthy horizons framework: a report to the Australian Health Ministers' Advisory Council', <http://www.ruralhealth.org.au/nrhapublic/publicdocs/hh/03_hhprogress.pdf>, viewed 28 May 2004.

Neuman, W.L 2000, *Social Research Methods: Qualitative and Quantitative Approaches*, 4th edn, Allyn and Bacon, Boston.

Newbold, S.K. 2002, 'FAQ about nursing informatics', *Nursing*, March.

New South Wales Ministerial Advisory Committee on Privacy and Health Information 2000, Report to the NSW Minister for Health: Panacea or Placebo? <http://www.health.nsw.gov.au/policy/gap/privacy/eprivacy.pdf>, viewed 15 May 2004.

New Zealand Ministry of Health 2000, *The New Zealand Health Strategy*, <http://www.moh.govt.nz/moh.nsf/f872666357c511eb4c25666d000c8888/a620173a2b7f179ecc256df700794563?OpenDocument>, viewed 10 April 2004.

New Zealand Ministry of Health 2004, New Zealand Health Information Service, <http://www.nzhis.govt.nz/>, viewed 6 October 2004.

New Zealand Ministry of Health 2004, *New Zealand Health Strategy*, online version, <http://www.moh.govt.nz/publications/nzhs>, viewed 30 September 2004.

Norris, A.C. 2002, 'Current trends and challenges in health informatics', *Health Informatics Journal*, California, vol. 8, pp. 205–13.

Nykanen, P. 2003, *On the Ontology of a Decision Support System in Health Informatics*, Idea Group Publishing, Hershey, PA.

O'Connor, P. 2003, 'Electronic medical records and diabetes care improvement: are we waiting for Godot?' <http://www.findarticles.com/p/articles/mi_m0CUH/is_3_26/ai_98880509>, viewed 11 February 2004.

Office of the Prime Minister 2004, 'A ten year plan to strengthen health care', Office of the Prime Minister, Ottawa <http://pm.gc.ca/eng/news.asp?id=260>, viewed 16 December 2004.

Office of the Surgeon General, United States Department of Health 2004, *Public Health Priorities*, <http://www.surgeongeneral.gov/publichealthpriorities.html#health>, viewed 30 July 2004.

O'Keefe, C., Greenfield, P. & Goodchild, A. 2004, 'A decentralised approach to electronic consent and health information access control', *Journal of Research and Practice in Information Technology*, vol. 37, <http://titanium.dstc.edu.au/papers/JRPIT_2004.pdf>, viewed 15 December 2004.

Openclinical 2001, 'AI Systems in Clinical Practice' <http://www.openclinical.org/aisp_help.html>, viewed August 2004.

Outram, D. 1995, *The Enlightenment*, Cambridge University Press, Cambridge.

Overby, S. 2002, 'How to win friends and influence users: the ability to handle tough users is a vital skill for CIOs, since the success of any enterprise wide implementation hinges on user adoption', *CIO*, September, vol. 15, no. 23, p. 1.

Patterson, V., Humphreys, J., Chua, R. 2003, 'Teleneurology by email', *Journal of Telemedicine and Telecare*, vol. 9, supplement 2, pp. 42–3.

Peisner, L. 2004, 'The virtual house call', *HomeCare Magazine*, vol. 27, no. 6, pp. 50–1.

Phillips, G. 2003, 'Guthrie cards', *Catalyst*, ABC, <http://www.abc.net.au/catalyst/stories/s867619.htm>, viewed 15 December 2004.

Pooley, E. 2002, 'Easing the high-tech transition: the secret to successful health technology integration isn't in the databases, but in how their users adapt to change', *Canadian Healthcare Manager*, September, vol. 9, no. 5, p. 19.

Protti, D. 2002, 'The EHR journey in the UK: a change in direction?' Nyborg, Denmark, <http://www.epj-observatoriet.dk/konference2002/konferenceslides/DenisProtti.pdf>, viewed 13 April 2004.

Ramnarayan, J. & Britto, J. 2002, 'Paediatric clinical decision support', *Archives of Disease in Childhood*, vol. 87, no. 5, pp. 361–2.

Raymond, E. 2000, 'The cathedral and the bazaar', <http://www.catb.org/~esr/writings/cathedral-bazaar/cathedral-bazaar/>, viewed 15 January 2004.

Richey, K. 2004, 'The ENIAC', <http://ei.cs.vt.edu/~history/ENIAC.Richey.HTML>, viewed 3 July 2004.

Rider, E. 2002, 'Telemedicine: the future is here', University of Nebraska, <http://communityprograms.unl.edu/html/pdf/HEF518.pdf>, viewed 11 January 2003.

Rogers, E. 1995, *Diffusion of Innovations*, 4th edn, The Free Press, New York.

Rola, M. 2003, 'Fully automated physicians' offices have become a security nightmare', *Technology in Government*, July/August, vol. 10, no. 7.

Rosenbaum, S., Hinderer, D., Scarborough, P. 1999, 'How usability engineering can improve clinical information systems', Usability Professionals' Association, <http://www.teced.com/PDFs/upa99sr.pdf>, viewed 16 December 2004.

Ruegger, M. & Johns, R. 1992, *Using Systems Theory in Social Work*, Open Learning Foundation Enterprises Ltd, London.

Russell, K. 2000, Health firms trail e-technology curve, Tennessean.com, <http://www.tennessean.com/sii/00/06/25/ehealth25.shtml>, viewed September 2004.

Russell, T., Buttrum, P., Wootton, R. & Hull, G. 2003, 'Low bandwidth physical rehabilitation for total knee replacement patients: preliminary results', *Journal of Telemedicine and Telecare*, vol. 9, supplement 2, pp. 15–19.

Saranummi, N., Korhonen, I., van Gils, M. & Kivisaari, S. 2001, 'Barriers limiting the diffusion of ICT for proactive and pervasive health care', *VTT Information Technology*, Tampere, Finland,<http://www.vtt.fi/tte/tte5/pdf/MEDICON_2001_Saranummi_et_al.pdf>, viewed 16 December 2004.

Savenstedt, S., Zingmark, K. & Sandman, PO. 2003, 'Video-phone communication with cognitively impaired elderly patients', *Journal of Telemedicine and Telecare*, vol. 9, supplement 2, pp. 52–3.

Schloeffel, P., 1998, 'Requirements for managing clinical information in integrated care', *Healthcare Review Online*, vol. 2, no. 12, <http://www.enigma.co.nz/hcro/website/index.cfm?fuseaction=articledisplay&FeatureID=54>, viewed 12 March 2003.

Schmit, S. & Appleby, J. 2004, 'Report to promote e-records for health care', *USA Today*, <http://www.usatoday.com/money/industries/health/2004-07-20-healthtech_x.htm>, viewed 20 August 2004.

Schoen, C., Blendon, R., DesRoches, M., Osborn, R., Raleigh, E., Huynh, P., Ho, A. & Zapert, K. 2003, 'Commonwealth Fund International Health Policy Survey of Hospital Executives', Summary Chartpack, <http://www.cmwf.org/usr_doc/2003_IHP_Survey_Chartpack.pdf>, viewed 23 June 2004.

Shahar, Y. 2001, 'Challenges in medical informatics: successes and failures', IMIA Invited Satellite Working Conference, cited by Wright, G. 2002, Centre for Health Informatics Research and Development, <http://www.chirad.org.uk/>, viewed 11 June 2004.

Shortliffe, E.H. 1989, 'Testing reality: the introduction of decision support technologies for physicians', *Methods of Information Medicine*, vol. 28, pp. 1–5.

Sintchenko, V., Westbrook, J., Tipper, S., Mathie, M. & Coiera, E. 2002, 'Electronic decision support activities in different healthcare settings in Australia', commissioned study published as Appendix A of *Electronic Decision Support for Australia's Health Sector, Report to Health Ministers by the National Electronic Decision Support Taskforce*, <http://www.openclinical.org/publicreportsDS.html>, viewed 11 March 2004.

Smith, J.D. 2004a, *Australia's Rural and Remote Health*, Tertiary Press, Croydon, Victoria.

Smith, R. 2004b, 'Can IT lead to radical redesign of health care?', Editor's Choice, *British Medical Journal*, 328, 15 May, <http://www.lmk.lu.se/pdf/15maj04.pdf>, viewed 30 May 2004.

Stone, E.M., Heinold, J.W. & Ewing, L.M. 2002, 'Accessing physician information on the Internet', The Commonwealth Fund, <http://www.cmwf.org/publications/publications_show.htm?doc_id=221298>, viewed 10 September 2004.

Sumner, M. 1999, 'Critical success factors in enterprise wide information management system projects', Special Interest Group on Computer Personnel Research, Annual Conference Proceedings of the 1999 ACM SIGCPR Conference on Computer Personnel Research, New Orleans, LA, pp. 297–303, <http://portal.acm.org/citation.cfm?id=299722>, viewed 15 January 2004.

Szolovits, P. (ed.) 1982, *Artificial Intelligence in Medicine*, Westview Press, Boulder, CO.

Talman, J.L. & Hasman, A. 2003, 'Medical informatics as a discipline at the beginning of the 21st century', in R. Haux and C. Kulikowski (eds), *Yearbook of Medical Informatics*, International Medical Informatics Association and Schattauer GmbH, Stuttgart, NY.

Tan, J.K.H & Hanna, J. 1994, 'Integrating Health Care with Information Technology: Knitting Patient Information Through Networking', *Health Care Management Review*, vol. 19, no. 2, pp. 78–80.

Tanriverdi, H. & Iacono, S. 1999, 'Diffusion of telemedicine: a knowledge barrier perspective', *Telemedicine Journal*, vol. 5, No. 3, pp. 223–44.

Taylor, C. 2002, 'Pathways to Professionalism in Health Informatics: Report on a One Day Conference and Workshop', <http://www.nhsia.nhs.uk/pdf/ukchip_pathways.pdf>, viewed 23 December 2003.

Teutsch, D., 2004, 'Sex-change patient's file put on the net', *Sydney Morning Herald*, <http://www.smh.com.au/articles/2004/06/05/1086377188047.html?from=storylhs>, viewed 13 December 2004.

Tolentino, H.D. 1999, 'Definitions of medical informatics', *Medical Informatics*, <http://www.veranda.com.ph/hermant/definitions.htm>, viewed 20 July 2002.

Trowbridge, R. & Weingarten, S. 2002, 'Chapter 53: Clinical decision support systems', in *Health Services/Technology Assessment Text*, US National Library of Medicine, <http://www.ncbi.nlm.nih.gov/books/bv.fcgi?rid=hstat1.section.62572>, viewed 17 December January 2003.

United Kingdom Department of Health 2001a, 'The expert patient: a new approach to chronic disease management for the 21st century', <http://www.dh.gov.uk/PublicationsAndStatistics/Publications/PublicationsPolicyAndGuidance/Publications PolicyAndGuidanceArticle/fs/en?CONTENT_ID=4006801&chk=UQCoh9>, viewed 15 July 2004.

United Kingdom Department of Health 2001b, 'Shifting gears', A report on the NHS Plan public consultation, <http://www.publications.doh.gov.uk/nhsplan/shiftinggears.htm#mod>, viewed 10 June 2004.

United Kingdom Department of Health News 2003, 'Every patient to get electronic patient record', <http://www.icesdoh.org/news.asp?ID=219>, viewed 16 December 2004.

United States Department of Health and Human Services 2004, Fact Sheet, *The Decade of Information Technology: Delivering Consumer-centric and Information-Rich Health Care*, <http://www.hhs.gov/news/press/2004pres/20040721.html>, viewed 2 July 2004.

van Krieken, R., Smith, P., Habibis, D., McDonald, K., Haralambos & M., Holborn, M. 2000, *Sociology: Themes and Perspectives*, 2nd edn, Longman, Melbourne.

Wachter, G. 2002, 'E-health lite: averting risks and laying the foundation', *Telemedicine Information Exchange*, <http://tie.telemed.org/news/features/ehealth02.asp>, viewed 12 February 2003.

Waegemann, P. 2003, 'EHR vs. CPR vs. EMR', *Healthcare Informatics*, <http://www.healthcareinformatics.com/issues/2003/05_03/cover_ehr.htm>, viewed 12 December 2003.

Walker, J. & Whetton, S. 2002, 'The diffusion of innovation: factors influencing the uptake of telehealth', *Journal of Telemedicine and Telecare*, vol. 8, supplement 3, pp. 73–5.

Watson, R.T. 2002, *Data management: Databases and Organisations*, 3rd edn, John Wiley & Sons, New York.

Whetton, S. 2002, The diffusion of an innovation: an investigation of the impact of innovation attributes, organisational characteristics and user characteristics on the adoption of health informatics education, Masters thesis, University of Tasmania, Launceston.

Wilkinson, D. & Blue, I. 2002, *The New Rural Health*, Oxford University Press, Melbourne.

Willcocks, S.G. 2004, 'Clinician managers and cultural context: comparisons between secondary and primary care', *Health Services Management Research*, February, vol. 17, no. 1, pp. 36–47.

Wilson, L. 1999, 'Computer-based expert assistance for radiologists', CD Rom: HIC99, Proceedings, August, Hobart.

Wootton, R., Blignault, I. & Cignoloi, J. 2003, 'A national survey of activity in Australian hospitals', *Journal of Telemedicine and Telecare*, vol. 9, supplement 2, pp. 73–5.

World Health Organization 2004, *World Health Report: Changing History*, WHO, Geneva<http://www.who.int/whr/2004/annex/topic/en/annex_5_en.pdf>, viewed 1 October 2004.

Wright, G. 2002, 'Health informatics', <http://www.chirad.org.uk/what+is+health+informatics.ppt#256,1,Health Informatics>, viewed 3 March 2004.

Yellowlees, P. 2000, *Your Guide to E-Health: Third Millennium Medicine on the Internet*, University of Queensland Press, Brisbane.

Index